To Ivan
sonhanc

Lloyd Percival

Coach and Visionary

I'm sorry for
our
mistake.
Thank you for you
help

Lloyd Percival
Coach and Visionary

by Gary Mossman

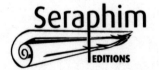

Seraphim
EDITIONS

The publisher wishes to express its appreciation to the Canadian Broadcasting
Corporation for quotes from the following radio and television programs: Sports
College of the Air, 1945; Assignment, 1958; Price of Hockey Stardom, 1961; Date
with Destiny; The Day It Is, 1968; Front Page Challenge, 1967; and Concern, 1974.

The publisher gratefully acknowledges the financial assistance of the Canada
Council for the Arts.

 Canada Council   **Conseil des Arts**
for the Arts   **du Canada**

Library and Archives Canada Cataloguing in Publication

Mossman, Gary, 1953-, author
    Lloyd Percival : coach and visionary / by Gary Mossman.

ISBN 978-1-927079-18-8 (pbk.)

    1. Percival, Lloyd, 1913-1974. 2. Athletic trainers--Canada--
Biography. 3. Coaches (Athletics)--Canada--Biography. 4. Fitness
Institute (Toronto, Ont.)--Biography. 5. Sports College (Radio program)--
Biography. 6. Physical fitness--Canada. I. Title.

GV697.P47M67 2013   796.092   C2013-905024-8

Editor: Kathryn McKeen
Design and Typography: Julie McNeill, McNeill Design Arts

Published in 2013 by
Seraphim Editions
54 Bay Street
Woodstock, ON
Canada N4S 3K9

Printed and bound in Canada

To my father who introduced me to the joys of
sport, and to his friend, Lloyd Percival.

Table of Contents

Preface   9

PART I: The Student 1913–1944

Childhood and Youth   17
The Odyssey   21

PART II: Sports College 'Head Coach' 1944–1964

CBC Sports College of the Air   33
Hockey   46
Track and Field   79
Other Sports   115
Research Studies, Publications and Government Policy   122
A Phoenix Rises in Don Mills   151
Sports College: The Final Years   161

PART III: The Guru 1964–1974

The Fitness Institute   169
1964 Tokyo Olympics   177
Sports Organizations and Individual Athletes   182
Drugs and Track and Field   186
George Chuvalo vs. Muhammed Ali   194
Lloyd Percival vs. COTFA   199
Final Retirement from Track and Field   216
Canada's First Cardiac Rehabilitation Program   235
The New Fitness Institute   237
Canada's High Priest of Physical Fitness   247
The Task Force Report on Sport for Canadians   249
Hockey Canada   257
The National Sport and Recreation Centre   260

The Coaching Association of Canada   262
The *sports & fitness Instructor*   270
ParticipACTION   275
Canadian Olympic Association and Game Plan '76'   278
Individual Athletes and Sports Associations   281
Hockey   297
Special Delivery and Rhythmics   310
A Fitness Institute Without Lloyd Percival   312
Goodbye Dear Coach   319

PART IV: Legacy

When Canada Was at Last Ready for Him   327
The Business of Fitness and the Health of a Nation   328
The 1976 Montreal Olympics   332
Government Policy   335
International Hockey and "The New NHL"   337
Coaching   342

Epilogue   345

Acknowledgements   346

Whoso would be a man must be a non-conformist.
RALPH WALDO EMERSON

By Courage to the Utmost
"SPORTS COLLEGE" MOTTO

Preface

"I'm a controversialist. People either swear by me,
or swear at me."

LLOYD PERCIVAL

DURING HIS EXTRAORDINARY CAREER as an athlete, a health and physical fitness expert and a media personality, but first and foremost as a coach, millions of Canadians swore by Lloyd Percival because he was a coach like no other coach Canada has ever seen. He not only instructed individual athletes and teams, he coached the coaches, and he shared his expertise with an entire nation. He did it personally and he did it through print, radio and television. For decades, a household name from coast-to-coast, Percival was one of the most successful and influential figures in Canadian sport during the years of profound change following WWII. He became a popular hero because he loved to speak his mind and the bane of the establishment because he insisted upon it.

Robert Fulford is one of those individuals who swore by Lloyd Percival. Fulford, one of Canada's most respected journalists and cultural observers of the second half of the twentieth century, met Percival in 1950 when Fulford was eighteen years old and had just landed his first job as a sports reporter for the *Globe and Mail*. Fulford quickly discovered that he was neither excited nor amused by "watching people play games," and has since become an unabashed critic of modern society's addiction to sport. While he honed his craft and awaited deliverance from the journalistic suburbs, Fulford had the great fortune to find Lloyd Percival, "hip deep in mediocrity, thoughtlessness and ignorance."

Percival's refusal to sit still for mediocrity and his belief that good enough was not good enough helped shape the young journalist's life. Even today, Fulford praises Percival in the same breath as he speaks of Canada's most famous cultural critic of the twentieth century, Marshall McLuhan. Like McLuhan, "Percival wanted to look at this thing people took for granted – he wanted to look at it in a structural and analytic way – he wanted to take it apart." During their lifetimes, both Percival and McLuhan were misunderstood and misrepresented because they were driven by one of McLuhan's favourite precepts: "There is absolutely no inevitability as long as there is a willingness to contemplate what is happening." Both men prodded and provoked, and looked beyond their narrow disciplines. Before interdisciplinary was even a word, Percival and McLuhan were seeking an integrated understanding of their universe, endeavouring to create a new science. Darlings of the media because they were so erudite and controversial, they were distrusted by establishment figures everywhere because, as McLuhan wrote, "The poet, the artist, the sleuth – whoever sharpens our perception tends to be antisocial; rarely "well adjusted," he cannot go along with currents and trends."

Lloyd Percival spent his entire adult life swimming against the current and challenging complacency wherever he found it. He was opinionated, arrogant, vociferous, confident, demanding, unyielding, and destined to become embroiled in controversy. He had an almost pathological need for self-promotion, an unwavering belief that he was right, a complete lack of patience with those who didn't share his beliefs, and he repeatedly became engaged in private skirmishes as well as in some that became all too public. Percival was also kind, generous, loyal and self-effacing; he inspired life-long loyalty from all who got to know him, and he was loved and deeply respected by all of the athletes he coached. The story of those years Percival spent confronting the status quo, fighting wave after wave of rejection of his unorthodox ideas, reveals much about Percival, the man and the coach, as well as about the times in which he lived.

Percival is best known as the author of *The Hockey Handbook* (1951). It has been read by millions of Canadians and, in print sixty years after it was written, remains one of the top selling hockey books in Canada; it may still be the best hockey instructional book ever written. Anatoly Tarasov used it to help the Soviet Union become a world hockey power, even though NHL coaches ignored it. European and American hockey coaches accepted Percival as the leading expert on Canadian hockey, but Canadian hockey experts thought that he was a quack. Percival's thirty year struggle with the powers that be in Canadian hockey and an understanding of the seminal role he played in the emergence of the "New NHL" in the twenty-first century is virtually unknown to Canadians.

Even less well known is that Percival's contribution to Canada's favourite sport is only the tip of the iceberg. From 1944 to 1964, as many as one million listeners tuned in to Percival's weekly "Sports College" radio program; his track and field clubs dominated every domestic track meet they entered, and he had his fingerprints on virtually all major sporting events involving Canadians between 1948 and 1976 including every Olympic, British Empire, and Pan-American Games, the 1966 Muhammad Ali/George Chuvalo fight, the triumphs of the Crazy Canuck skiers, the Bannister/Landy Miracle Mile, and the 1972 Canada/Russia Hockey Series. In spite of this success, Percival was never selected to coach a national team, and his contributions were regularly discounted by his peers.

Percival was as interested in rebuilding as he was in deconstructing because he was a 'scientist' as well as a 'poet'. We see this in the innovative training programs Percival used to help develop many of the greatest names in Canadian sport history, first through "Sports College" and, after 1963, at The Fitness Institute, the first modern fitness and athletic training facility this side of the "Iron Curtain" where Olympic medalists Ken Lane and Don Hawgood (1952), Roger Jackson (1964), John Wood (1976), Kathy Kreiner (1976), Toller Cranston (1976) and Steve Podborski (1980) all trained under Percival prior to winning their Olympic medals. Hockey Hall of

Fame members Gordie Howe, Terry Sawchuck, Ted Lindsay, Red Kelly, Frank Mahovlich and Dick Duff were amongst the hundreds of hockey players he worked with. Boxer, George Chuvalo; cyclist, Jocelyn Lovell; water-ski legend, George Athans Jr.; divers, Beverly Boys, Nancy Robertson and Cindy Shatto; skiers, 'Jungle' Jim Hunter and Judy Crawford; football players, Jim Corrigal and Dave Raimey; golfers, George Knudson and Al Balding; fastball pitcher, Bob Domik; tennis players, Peter Burwash and Harry Fauquier; FI driver, George Eaton; equestrians, Jim Day and Terry Liebel; track and field athletes, Rich Ferguson and Nancy McCredie; and figure skaters, Val and Sandra Bezic, all dominated their sports in Canada; most were amongst the best in the world. Some of these athletes worked closely with Percival for years; others spent only a short time at The Fitness Institute, but all of them owe some degree of their success to the institute's cutting edge training programs, the psychological preparation and the intuitive coaching of Lloyd Percival. Several athletes say they owe Percival much, much more.

Percival also led a relentless crusade to incorporate sport and fitness into government policy. He published brief after brief, detailing not only that which was wrong with Canada's athletic endeavours but also exactly what to do to rectify the situation. He was a thorn in the side of Canada's public servants for more than thirty years before his conviction that sport was a legitimate part of Canada's cultural mosaic found a place in the 1969 *Task Force on Sport for Canadians*. In spite of his significant influence on the flood of government policy that followed, it would be thirty years after Percival's death that his vision was fully embraced. Throughout it all he worried about the health of the average Canadian. The numerous studies and booklets he published to help people eat and exercise their way to more enjoyable and fulfilling lives contained nutritional information and advice that was years, and sometimes decades, ahead of its time.

Lloyd Percival was a visionary, and his work was ground-breaking. Robert Fulford compares him to Marshall McLuhan. Dr. Paul McGoey, chief surgeon at Scarborough General Hospital stated, "like Banting and Best, he (Percival) was self-taught and we must respect his single-mindedness of purpose and devotion of his whole life to physical fitness." Douglas Fisher, MP, lobbyist, journalist and, for twenty years, sport's most influential voice in Ottawa called Percival, "surely the most indefatigable missionary Canadian sport has ever had." Fisher also believed that Percival and Glenn Gould had something in common: "a bravery – a description and a prescription for change." McLuhan, Banting, Best and Gould occupy prominent positions in the pantheon of great Canadians; their careers and accomplishments are part of school curriculums across the country. Lloyd Percival has been all but forgotten.

PART I

The Student 1913–1944

Childhood and Youth

LLOYD ALWYN PERCIVAL WAS BORN IN TORONTO on June 3, 1913, to James and Lydia Ann (nee Curphey) Percival. Lloyd was the middle child, preceded by Gordon in 1909, and followed by Alan in 1921. James Percival was a former athlete who worked as an executive for the clothing department at Eaton's Department Stores; Lydia had trained to be a concert pianist. Amongst Lloyd's earliest recollections was "being trundled off to various sports events" by his British-born parents, while music also provided a wellspring of joy and comfort throughout his life.

The Percival family's first home on Pricefield Road in Toronto's affluent Rosedale neighbourhood was next door to the Toronto Tennis Club where the three boys would pass much of their youth. The family later moved to a slightly larger home at 30 Nanton Street in South Rosedale. For a few years, Lloyd attended Havergal College, the private girl's school favoured by Toronto's elite, at a time when young boys were also taught there. Lloyd gained most of his early education, as did his brothers, at Rosedale's Whitney Public School where he won the Hatch Trophy awarded to the school's best all-round athlete.

During those years, Rosedale was still "the heartland of English Canada – with a way of life that was comfortable, cultured and staunchly British." It was, therefore, one of the centres of the British-rooted sporting culture that had been transplanted to Canada in the 19th Century. The first sports that Lloyd and his brothers excelled at were the same ones their parents had grown up with in England – tennis, soccer, cricket and rugby. Lloyd joined the Yorkshire Society Cricket Club when he was only thirteen years old. At sixteen, he was a mainstay of the club and was one of five players honoured with trophies at the club's annual general meeting in December 1929. After winning a number of local tournaments, Lloyd reached the finals of the 1929 Canadian Junior Tennis Championships before losing to reigning United States Junior Champion, Frankie Parker. A few years later, Lloyd and Alan played in the national doubles finals.

It was not only the physical nature of the sports of his forefathers that attracted Percival. He also appreciated the ideology of the British and their gentlemanly attitude to sport. "Fair play, physical hardiness, physical and mental well-being, courage, endurance, teamwork, efficiency, self-restraint, innovation, competitiveness, and respect for others" were believed to be ingrained in the individual through participation in sport and were considered essential to success in the modern age. They were remnants of the Victorian love affair with Classical Greece, the ideals of the ancient Olympic Games, and the modern sporting traditions that the British believed were their legitimate offspring. We have good reason for being more cynical today, but in his youth Percival was surrounded by people who were convinced that these sporting ideals could be a powerful force for good in society.

A pugnacious individualism and a deep respect for the non-conformist also marked Percival's character from a very young age. For this he acknowledged a debt to his father, who imparted to him a healthy combination of envy and distrust for the tremendously successful American sporting system and the manner in which it promoted individualism and class equality. Craving more than the genteel sports of Rosedale, Percival crossed Yonge Street's sociological divide and joined the Maitlands Athletic Club of Cottingham Square, where "the rich kid from Rosedale with the grey flannel shorts and the sissy name" proved he could hold his own with some of the best hockey and lacrosse players in Toronto. Percival loved the tough physical nature and the free flowing creativity of the quintessential Canadian sports. At the Maitlands' Athletic Club, he also learned firsthand about the social levelling that sport could engender. Most importantly, Percival learned how to fight, both with his body and with his mind.

Once Percival had finished using his fists to prove that he belonged with the youth of Cottingham Square, he entered the ring and developed a lifelong love of boxing – a rare photo of Lloyd at no more than ten years of age, wearing boxing trunks and gloves and striking a classic boxing pose, displays the visage of a champion. Percival tasted defeat in the ring only once in twenty-eight amateur fights – to Vince Glionna at the 1928 Canadian Olympic Trials. Glionna won the bantamweight division and finished in a tie for fifth place at the Olympics in Amsterdam, but it was the fifteen year old "baby-faced" Percival, still too young to be named to the Olympic team, who captured the imagination of the crowd. Lou Marsh, the *Toronto Star* reporter, after whom the trophy awarded annually to Canada's top athlete is named, described him as "a little pink-skinned blond with long taffy coloured locks ... fussy name ... and flossy get-up ... (who) waded into Glionna as if the only Glionna he ever heard of was a fiddler." Although Percival was fairly beaten, the crowd "jeered" when the decision was announced. His "grit, courage and fearlessness" had impressed everyone. According to Marsh, this, combined with an "unexpected cleverness" made him a "comer – make no mistake about that."

Along with boxing, lacrosse, hockey, cricket, and tennis, Percival also excelled at wrestling, gymnastics, table tennis, football, baseball, and track and field. In spite of the success he enjoyed in all of these sports, it was his failure to win the top prize at the 1929 Canadian Junior Tennis Championships that proved to be the pivotal event in Percival's young life. For most any other Canadian teenager, losing to the best junior tennis player in the United States would have been disappointing but not catastrophic. Percival was no ordinary teenager. He immediately went to Parker's famous coach, Mercer Beasley, and demanded to know how he, the "stronger, faster and better-conditioned" athlete, had lost? Beasley's answer was succinct. "Coaching" was the difference.

Percival returned home to reflect upon the defeat and Beasley's response to his question. He'd never really been coached, and the more he thought about it, the more Percival realized that he had no idea where in Canada he could find good coaching. There were plenty of men, and a few women, who volunteered their time at pools, gymnasiums, ice rinks and athletic fields across the country – usually former athletes who passed on some of the lessons learned during their own sporting careers. But it was rare to find one who had any knowledge of the new "sport sciences" which were emerging in the United States and in Europe. Percival concluded that his situation was neither unique nor inevitable, and his "willingness to contemplate what was happening," to himself as well as to other athletes in Canada transformed a search for an explanation for his personal setback into a desire to understand and become a part of the solution. Lloyd Percival decided to become a coach.

Since there were no schools in North America that offered regular courses on coaching and no well-trodden path for him to follow, Percival concluded that he would have to travel. Fortunately, his parents were very supportive. "OK," he remembered his father saying, "you want to be a coach. Go ahead and be a good one. I'll back you." The teenager embarked on an odyssey which lasted more than a decade. While his studies took him to places he could not have imagined in the beginning, his was not a voyage managed by capricious gods. Percival plotted a course carefully designed to search out the essence of coaching and all that it entailed.

The Odyssey

PERCIVAL'S FIRST STOP WAS NEW YORK CITY and the offices of *The New York Times*, where John Kieran, the best-known sportswriter of his era, wrote his daily column, "Sports of the Times." Kieran was much more than a sportswriter. He was a poet, a Shakespearean scholar and head of the American National Audubon Society. Eclectic and well-rounded, Kieran was atypical to the world of sport, but he was the type of person to whom Percival would be drawn to throughout his life. Kieran advised Percival to "play every game he could," and to "learn to coach them, referee and write about them." Most importantly, he insisted that Percival "study under famous instructors."

The first mentor Kieran suggested for Percival was Knute Rockne, University of Notre Dame football coach from 1917 to 1931. Rockne is best remembered as the inventor of the forward pass and for his "win one for the Gipper" speech, but Rockne contributed much more to the development of modern sport. Because of his openness and curiosity, the famous "Notre Dame shift" was inspired by the precision and timing of a Broadway chorus line. He designed equipment that was less bulky yet offered more protection; he was the first to take his team across the country to foster the great college football rivalries of today; he employed psychological weapons like no coach before him, and as "the first entrepreneurial coach," used sportswriters and radio to aggressively promote himself and the school. Rockne was the Notre Dame Athletic Director, business manager, ticket distributor, and track and field manager. He also wrote a weekly newspaper column and authored three books. During the summer, Rockne ran coaching camps at Notre Dame's South Bend, Indiana campus where he mentored many of the best young coaches in America and, in the summer of 1930, one wide-eyed, young Canadian.

Throughout his life, Percival kept a painting of Knute Rockne above his desk and often credited his mentor with furnishing the cornerstones of his coaching philosophy, the framework he built for them, and his appreciation for the all-encompassing nature of his vocation. It was the manner in which Rockne approached the needs of each athlete on an individual basis, however, that most impressed Percival. As simple as that sounds, it was a concept that was foreign to most coaches at that time, remained so for decades, and still eludes many coaches today.

Rockne's coaching career was tragically cut short by a fatal aeroplane crash the following year – the same year that Percival`s coaching career began. In the spring of 1931, Percival convinced the Yorkshire Cricket Club executive to name him coach of the club's entry in the new Toronto Cricket Council Junior League, even though he was yet to celebrate his eighteenth birthday. When the cricket season was over, Percival became coach of the National Sea Fleas midget hockey team. Lou Marsh, Harry 'Red' Foster, founder of Canadian Special Olympics, and future Maple Leaf owner, Harold Ballard, operated the hockey program on behalf of the outboard racing division of the National Yacht Club. Marsh's earlier impressions of the "grit, courage and fearlessness" of Percival the boxer undoubtedly influenced the decision to install the eighteen year old behind a bench stocked with some of Toronto's best sixteen and seventeen year old hockey players.

In spite of his age, Percival was able to gain the trust of a group of players that included Paul McGoey, who traded his skates for a scalpel and became a leading orthopaedic specialist and chief surgeon at Scarborough General Hospital, along with future Hockey Hall of Fame member Bobby Bauer. The Sea Fleas went undefeated that year. What is more remarkable is that they scored 271 goals, while allowing only four against them. Two of the games were played against the Toronto Marlboro's midget team. The Sea Fleas won those games,

5-0 and 11-0. In the latter game, goalie Art Childs "became so bored and lonely that he sent out for a hot dog and a carton of coffee, which he consumed while leaning nonchalantly against his goal." This infuriated Toronto Marlboro and Maple Leaf owner, Conn Smythe, who reportedly confronted Percival after the game. Percival offered the same kind of coaching expertise for Smythe's teams, but Smythe declined. This was the first, but would not be the last, time that Percival and the Smythe family locked horns.

Percival coached the Sea Fleas for only one season, choosing instead to return again and again to the United States in search of more secrets to good coaching. He spent two years at a high school in Omaha, Nebraska, studying journalism and competing in baseball, football, gymnastics, and track and field; he studied exercise physiology for one semester at Springfield College in Massachusetts (with an emphasis on testing and measurement), and attended clinics and camps run by American coaching luminaries Lou Little and Dean Cromwell. Little had brought Georgetown and Columbia University football teams to national prominence. Like Rockne, he is remembered not only for developing great football teams but also for building a great athletic program. Cromwell, the University of Southern California (USC) track and field coach, was nicknamed "Maker of Champions" because he coached ten Olympic Gold Medal winners between 1912 and 1948 – at least one at each Olympiad. Percival often stated that Cromwell had invited him to stay on as a coach at USC but that he had declined.

Since Percival couldn't gain a personal audience with every sports and physical fitness expert in the world, he did the next best thing and wrote to them. In 1934, Percival began mailing questionnaires designed to uncover "the best techniques and knowledge available." By the end of the decade, he had sent out 1,800 questionnaires and 1,100 athletes and coaches throughout the world had replied. The understanding of athletes and athletics which Percival acquired through this correspondence was invaluable as he evolved a philosophy of sport and coaching. It also provided him with a list of contacts – a sort of international sports and fitness database – which would be integral to Percival becoming the best educated and best informed Canadian coach of his generation.

In order to finance his travel, Percival played a ukulele and sang in a group called the Varsity Entertainer. He also "picked up pin money writing a certain horrible type of verse," under the pen name, Lou Allen. For the most part, however, Percival followed Kieran's advice when selecting part-time jobs. He sold sporting goods and wrote sports pulp fiction for an American magazine while continuing his peripatetic career as an athlete.

After winning a regional Golden Gloves title in 1930, Percival turned down an offer to become a professional boxer and his amateur career soon ended when a head butt left him totally blind for three months and partially blind in one eye for the rest of his life. During the decade of the 1930s, Percival would also reject a professional contract offer from Teddy Oke's Millionaires of the International Hockey League along with offers to play professional cricket in Europe. Instead, he played and refereed a number of amateur sports in Toronto, coached and learned about administration.

Cricket was the sport Percival played most often and for the most years. He was one of the best batsmen in Canada and almost as dominating a bowler. He and his brother, Gordon, were stars of the Yorkshire Cricket Club XI. When Alan came of age, the three brothers starred at the Rosedale Cricket Club. In the beginning, Gordon was the superior player. Later, Alan's tremendous natural athletic ability often shone through, but Lloyd usually dominated not only his brothers but also many a cricket match. In later years, Percival initiated a "Sports College" study that found that the majority of "championship athletes" were middle children. After consulting with psychologists, he concluded that middle children were successful in sports, as well as in other pursuits, because they possessed a "compulsion to succeed and win approval." This was the result of their having "to fight for attention" that was more naturally afforded to their siblings.

Lloyd was a member of representative cricket sides that Ontario sent to Quebec in 1930 and 1935; he was on the Eastern Canada XI that toured Western Canada in 1934; he played against England's famed Marylebone Cricket Club in Montreal in 1937 and was still a tower of strength in 1945 when an Ontario side travelled to up-state New York to challenge "Headley's Eleven" led by George Headley, "the Black Bradman" of the West Indies. Lloyd's finest moment, and one of the most cherished memories in his sporting life, came when he and Gordon represented Canada on a tour of England in 1936. Lloyd was first wicket when the Canadian team scored an unprecedented victory over Marylebone at the "hallowed ground of Lords" on July 25, 1936.

Instead of returning home at the end of the tour, Percival headed for Berlin where the 1936 Olympics were being held. He was struck by the pageantry and the politicization of the Games, as well as by the remarkable performances of Jesse Owens. But it was the disappointing showing of the Canadian team that made the greatest impression on the young Canadian. The nine medals Canada brought home were a far cry from the fifteen won in both 1928 and 1932, and the drop-off was most notable in the marquee sport of track and field. Athletes from all over the world were jumping higher, running faster and making huge strides in all sports, while Canadians were standing still. Hitler's Germany was the first nation to make a concerted effort to use sport to enhance its international reputation, but Percival predicted that it would not be the last. He believed that any country interested in keeping pace would have to create an environment in which athletes could flourish, and he returned home determined to help establish an infrastructure in Canada that would facilitate successful athletic endeavours.

Percival's initial contribution came in the form of correspondence with former English Captain, D.R. Jardine, concerning ways of improving the quality of cricket played in Canada. Soon, Percival was also operating the Rosedale Sports School where he offered instruction in all manner of sport, and he was writing a weekly column for the *Toronto Star* titled, "Comment from the Coach," but Percival's most ambitious project was the proposal for a national sports organization that he began preparing for the federal government. Percival often said that the seeds for a national sports organization in Canada were planted by Knute Rockne in 1930, but it was the 1936 Olympics and a conversation in 1937 with another exceptional American sports personality, Ted Husing, from whom Percival learned the finer points of sports broadcasting which enabled Percival to complete the framework for "Sports Club," the national sports information service that he envisaged being broadcast over the radio. Percival was granted a meeting in Ottawa with the Minister of Pensions and Health, Ian McKenzie. He came away empty-handed, having been informed by the minister that it was not practical for the government to get involved in such matters.

Undaunted, Percival continued with his sports school, his newspaper column and his education. The contacts he had made through his letter writing campaign and his trip to England and Germany in 1936 led Percival to return to Europe before the end of the decade. He spent one year studying combined physical education and athletic science at Loughborough College (now Loughborough University), England's "premier university for sport development, research and education." In the 1930s, it was a technical college and Captain F.A.M. Webster who "had an international reputation in sport and physical training as a writer, instructor, player and scientist," and was Head of the College School of Athletics, Games and Physical Training. Percival's autobiographical accounts also make reference to time spent studying at King's College in London and the Sokol Institute in Prague, Czechoslovakia.

When Canada entered the war in 1939, priorities changed for everyone. The damage Percival had incurred to his eye in his last boxing match left him unfit for military service. In later years, he told some people that he worked for Special Services during WWII, but the truth was undoubtedly less exotic than he made it sound. Besides devoting time to coaching cricketers at RAF airbases and after he had started "Sports College of the Air" near the end of the war producing two hour sports quiz shows which were then portioned into fifteen minute packages and aired at Canadian bases overseas, Percival continued to play cricket, run the Rosedale Sports School and write his *Toronto Star* column.

The "Comment from the Coach" column brought Percival correspondence from all across Canada and led to an announcement in the *Toronto Star* on October 19, 1940, that it was being expanded into a unique new service called "Sports Club." Percival was also doing a Friday night game show on CFRB radio station in Toronto called "Mental Athletics" in which listeners were rewarded with cash if they could answer the tough sports questions he prepared each week. In January or February 1941, "Sports Club" and "Mental Athletics" coalesced into "Sports College" and found a home at radio station CKOC in Hamilton. He didn't have the government backing he had hoped for, but Percival was finally set to realize his goal of bringing sports and fitness instruction to a mass audience. First, however, two significant events in Percival's personal life profoundly affected his future.

Lloyd's father, James Percival, died suddenly of heart failure while he was in his early fifties. His death was consistent with a family history of heart problems which would be a source of concern to all three of the Percival children; it certainly contributed to Lloyd's life-long interest in health and nutrition, and probably was a factor in him aggressively pursuing his dream at this time.

The second event that dramatically changed Percival's life, and impacted upon everything he attempted thereafter, occurred in 1940 when Lloyd met Dorothy Elizabeth Macdonell – first, in the revolving door of the CBC building then upstairs when he discovered that she was answering an advertisement for secretarial help on a program that Percival was preparing. Dorothy was a fine tennis player and a national calibre fencer. She had followed Percival's career through the newspaper and thought that "working for him would be interesting." There was an immediate attraction and a short courtship. People were telling Percival and his bride-to-be that a radio version of "Sports Club" was a fine idea, but there was no one willing to back up their speeches with money. When the couple heard of the opportunity at CKOC in Hamilton, Dorothy convinced Lloyd that they should forego a honeymoon and use their money to buy time on the radio. For their savings, "Sports Club" renamed "Sports College" received one-half hour of weekly airtime for six months. Lloyd and Dorothy were married on February 3, 1941. They moved into the house on Nanton Street with Lloyd's mother and his two brothers, commuting to and from Hamilton for the radio broadcast.

Every Thursday night at 7:00 o'clock, Lloyd and his brother, Alan, offered coaching advice and answered questions sent in by listeners; occasionally they interviewed sports personalities. They were supported by Dorothy and whatever secretarial help they could afford. "Sports College" lived on after the Percivals' savings ran out with the help of income generated by advertising and promotions including revenue from a weekly cartoon featuring "Ace Percival, the world's most versatile athlete." The cartoon, sponsored by a breakfast food company, appeared in newspapers from 1943 until 1946 when Percival withdrew his support due to the possibility of conflict of interest; the moniker 'Ace' Percival, however, stuck with him for the rest of his life. By 1944, "Sports College" boasted 22,000 members; however, Percival was convinced that the program was worthy of a national platform. He also believed that without the money generated by a much larger audience, he could not produce the kind of material and provide the level of instruction that Canadians should have been receiving.

Percival was still convinced that the federal government was the best agent for any national fitness program, and in 1943, he had reason to believe that they would be more receptive to his ideas than had been the case in 1936. Of a total population of little more than twelve million people, almost one million Canadians served in WWII. Of those recruited, a full 33% were pronounced unfit for military service. As a result, the National Physical Fitness Act (NPFA) had been passed by the House of Commons and the National Council on Physical Fitness

(NCPF) established, with Ian Eisenhardt, former leader of British Columbia's "Pro Rec Movement," as director. Although the NPFA stressed "that total fitness must originate at home, the church, the school and the community," Percival believed that "Sports College" could be included in its mandate. In 1944, brief in hand, he headed back to Ottawa only to be quickly dismissed for a second time. The reality was that NPFA and the NCPF were fraught with confusion from the beginning. Unable to decide exactly what their mandate was and forced to co-operate with the provinces in some manner yet known, the members of the NCPF were in no position to work with Percival, and the government was not about to initiate any other project involving sport and fitness.

The CBC had always been Percival's first choice as a broadcaster for "Sports College" and he had twice auditioned tapes of the thirty-minute programme. Not only had the CBC turned him down, "Sports College's" days at CKOC were said to be numbered. The future of Percival's dream looked bleak until the Canadian National Council of Y.M.C.A.'s came to the rescue in 1944. At the Annual Meetings, held in Montreal between June 2nd and 6th of its centennial year, the National Council made recommendations for improving its delivery of education to the youth of Canada, creating better access to "communities or urban neighbourhoods not now reached by the Association," and finding ways to "co-operate with such bodies as the National Film Board, the Canadian Youth Commission and the Canadian Broadcasting Company." Percival's ambitions for "Sports College" were a perfect fit. A meeting took place later in June between Percival and William R. Cook, program director for the National Council of Y.M.C.A.s. That led to a meeting with Ernie Bushnell, Director General of Programs at the CBC. When Percival was finally convinced that a fifteen-minute format would be more effective, "Sports College of The Air" was born.

A standing committee was appointed "to be responsible for directing Y.M.C.A. "Sports College" … as a regular department of the National Council." Chairman of the committee was J. Ardagh

Scythes, a prominent Y.M.C.A. layman. Cook was named Executive Director, and Lloyd Percival was "Coach." On July 12, the committee met for the first time and Percival was presented with a contract that stated Lloyd Percival "is the sole proprietor of a broadcasting program known as "National "Sports College" and "the Y.M.C.A. has agreed to engage the services of Percival in conducting a Y.M.C.A. "Sports College" through co-operation and collaboration with the Canadian Broadcasting Corporation." The contract was set for one year, with the Y.M.C.A. having "the option of renewing this Agreement for two further periods of one year each." The Y.M.C.A. allocated office space on the eighth floor of the Hermant Building on Dundas Square in downtown Toronto and agreed to give Percival six months' notice prior to terminating their arrangement. The Y.M.C.A. accepted responsibility "for all organization and expenses" except broadcasting and set an initial budget for one year at $14,968.50, of which $4,500 was to be paid to Cook as Executive Director and $3,900 to Percival for:

Preparation of script for weekly broadcasts
Weekly narration
Preparing Special Bulletins, training schedules, etc.
Securing guest stars for broadcasts
And use of the name "Sports College"

Percival agreed to "faithfully and diligently serve the Y.M.C.A. and in all his relationships to the said Y.M.CA. "Sports College" to be governed by the aims and objectives and statement of purpose of the Y.M.C.A."

The space provided by the Y.M.C.A. was never enough for Percival. The family home at 30 Nanton Street was sold and a larger property purchased around the corner at 12 Glen Road. Lloyd, Dorothy and "Sports College" moved in upstairs, while his mother and two brothers occupied the downstairs. Alan married and moved out a few years later, but Gordon stayed on until, like his father, he died of a massive coronary while only in his fifties. The odyssey was over. Lloyd Percival was home.

PART II
Sports College 'Head Coach' 1944–1964

CBC Sports College of the Air

At 12:15 PM, on July 22, 1944, heard coast-to-coast for the first time on the CBC were the words:

> And now it's time for Sports College of the Air, a non-profit public service dedicated to raising the standards of health, physical fitness and sports efficiency.

Immediately afterwards there was an opening fanfare from C. J. Gilbert's Spirit of Youth March. For almost twenty years, each "Sports College" broadcast would begin this way and would follow the same simple formula. As the music faded out, Bill Bessey, in one of those distinguished mid-Atlantic voices cultivated by CBC announcers of the day, continued:

> The Canadian Broadcasting Corporation, in co-operation with the National Council of Y.M.C.A.s, presents Sports College of the Air. Attention young Canadians, once again it's time for the sports-minded members of Canada's only college of sports knowledge to gather round their radios to continue their studies of sport, which are expertly designed to help them become better athletes, perhaps even stars.

Bessey would then introduce the line-up for that particular broadcast and turn it over to the day's host. In the early days, this was usually Alan Percival; in later years it was always Lloyd or his associate, Doug MacLennan. The host would continue:

Hello Sports College members in Canada and the
United States. Welcome to Sports College session
number one.

Each program was jam-packed with information on amateur and
professional sports. The cause, treatment and prevention of sports
injuries were also regular topics on "Sports College," as were issues
of general health and fitness. As time passed, nutrition also became a
common theme. In almost every session, one of the "Sports College"
staff would interview "Head Coach, Lloyd Percival," from a script
Percival had written. This allowed Percival to impart knowledge in
a less didactic manner than if he had simply lectured. The pace was
brisk, but measured; the language clear and informal. There was
an air of familiarity, especially from Lloyd who had a real gift for
radio. He came across like everyone's wise but hip uncle; the one
you would listen to because he made it clear that he was a voice of
authority and knew what he was talking about but who didn't lecture
to you the way your father did.

The programs were never dull or dry, and Percival frequently
spiced them up with celebrity interviews. In the early years, the
majority of the guests were hockey players including Syl Apps,
Gordie Howe, Terry Sawchuck and Bobby Bauer. Bauer was featured
twice, in 1944 and 1945. In his second interview, the Boston Bruins
star delighted his host by informing the audience that "the season
that did me the most good is the season with the National Sea Fleas
coached by Lloyd Percival"; however, the range of interviews was as
diverse as the subjects Percival explored and included baseball star
Ernie Banks, heavyweight boxing champion Jack Dempsey, and two-
time Olympic gold medal pole vaulter, 'Reverend' Bob Richards, the
first athlete to be pictured on a Wheaties cereal box. The guest was
usually tied to the theme of the show and the theme was generally
a sport people were playing and watching at that particular time of
year. These discussions might also relate to recent "Sports College"
publications. Percival and the other on-air staff devoted part of each

program to soliciting memberships and informing members about the printed material that was available.

Each "Sports College" session ended the same way. The host would preview the following week's line-up before signing off with the "Sports College" motto:

Keep Fit, Work Hard, Play Fair and Live Clean.

"Sports College" was an immediate success and the audience grew exponentially. After just six broadcasts, 2,439 pieces of mail had been received from nine provinces and five American states. One of the essay writing contests that Percival used to attract new members produced 18,000 letters in one week alone. In June 1946, Cook reported that the program was still receiving as many as 10,000 letters per week and that the total listening audience was between 750,000 and 1,000,000 per episode. Considering that the program was primarily directed at boys and young men, was broadcast in an era when many adult males in Canada still worked a six day week and when the total population was less than thirteen million, it is clear that "Sports College" was an unparalleled success. Saturday Night magazine proclaimed it, "probably the most potent and popular health and sport skill building medium for youth on this continent."

People today still remember things that they learned from listening to Percival's Saturday broadcasts more than fifty years ago. Furthermore, Percival was a master of communication who intuitively knew, long before we read about it in academic journals, that simply hearing these things once over the radio did not ensure that they would be absorbed. He began exploring other mediums – film was on the agenda, but print came first.

For the first few years the publications were free – the quantity and quality truly impressive. Any boy (in the beginning the show was only directed at young males) in Canada or the United States who wrote in for a membership was eligible to receive the plethora of publications. Percival later boasted of having written three million words in "Sports College's" first year alone. Over the years, he would gain a well-deserved reputation for hyperbole, but if you look at the vast array of pamphlets, bulletins and scripts turned out by "Sports College," you can see that Percival wasn't far off the mark.

The initial publication, *How to Play Better Baseball*, released on Aug 30, 1944, was the first in a Playbetter series, which would include titles on hockey, football and basketball as well as *How to Build a Better Body* and *How to be a Better Coach*. That first booklet was an eight-page leaflet and the second in the series, *How to Play Better Hockey*, contained seventeen pages, but Percival soon decided to replace them with something more substantial. In the fall of 1945, he published a forty-nine page edition of *How to Play Better Baseball* and a fifty page version of *How to Play Better Hockey*. These Playbetter booklets were brilliantly conceived and represent a landmark in the history of sports instruction. Professional coach, Carl Bennett, stated that *How to Play Better Basketball* was "the best book on basketball (he had) ever seen" and arranged for the book to be distributed throughout the high schools of Indiana, the hotbed of basketball in the United States. Since hockey is Canada's sport, however, *How to Play Better Hockey* proved to be the most important volume in the series.

Almost everything Percival would introduce to the hockey world during his lifetime was explored in the six chapters of this surprisingly comprehensive booklet. Along with advice on shooting, skating, defensive play, goaltending, team tactics and strategy, Percival advised NHL teams to hire assistant coaches to teach different positions and skills and to take notes during games. He even suggested having one of them act as a spotter up in the stands and report to the coach between periods. Assistant coaches for the defence, goalies and special teams – some of whom watch the game from the press box – are commonplace in the NHL today but in 1945, Percival was speaking a language foreign to NHL coaches. He would still be trying to get through to them in 1969 when he reiterated:

> A coach can't expect to be an expert on everything
> from his vantage behind the bench. He should have
> assistants who concern themselves with specialized
> facets of the game … like in football where the
> head coach has assistants.

It wasn't until the 1980s that NHL coaches understood what Percival was talking about and began hiring assistant coaches.

Jack Adams, General Manager of the Detroit Red Wings, gave the book to his players but was not about to spend his money hiring extra coaches. Lester Patrick, one of the great innovators and pioneers in the history of professional hockey, was also impressed by the book and said, "… there doesn't appear to be a single fundamental that has been overlooked." While Patrick's admiration was not sufficient for him to introduce many of Percival's radical ideas to his New York Ranger team, he gave a copy of the book to Thomas A. Lockhart, President of the Amateur Hockey Association (AHA) of the United States. Lockhart ordered four hundred copies and distributed them to every member of the AHA. The majority within the inner circle of the NHL, however, reacted like Toronto Maple Leaf's coach, Clarence 'Hap' Day, who called *How to Play Better Hockey* "a lot of bunkum."

The unprecedented quantity and quality of the contents of the Playbetter publications were almost superseded by the singularity of the presentation. Each booklet measured only three and a half inches by two inches. Although 30,000 words were squeezed onto fifty pages of *How to Play Better Hockey*, it is neither cramped nor daunting to read. Unlike a standard-sized book or even a paperback, these booklets could be tucked into a coach or player's breast or jacket pocket.

Along with the Playbetter series, Percival and "Sports College" produced smaller booklets on *How to Train for Hockey* and *How to Improve at Track and Field*. There was also a series of Bulletins, each of which contained "ten important secrets of success" for a different sport, as well as General Bulletins on subjects as diverse as: *How to be a Better Referee and Umpire*; *Swimming and Water Safety Hints* and *Does Prayer help in Sport*. Finally, there was a series of short, Helpful Hints pamphlets on a dozen different sports, as well as on *Purchasing and Caring for Equipment* and *Recognition and Treatment of Injuries*.

All of these publications were produced within the first two years of operation. A truly impressive library of sports knowledge became available to anyone who was a "Sports College" member and who paid four cents per publication to cover the costs of postage and handling.

The CBC and "Sports College" reaped unexpected rewards from the overnight success of "Sports College." For the Y.M.C.A. that success was a double-edged sword. The program was a marvellous vehicle for the Christian mission of the Y.M.C.A. Cook reported that "without preaching religion it promotes ideas and activities which tend to develop unity of purpose and training in active co-operation among youth"; Cook even claimed a scriptural origin for the "Sports College" motto. Since seventy per cent of the "Sports College" audience lived in rural communities where there was no Y.M.C.A., the program also fulfilled the National Council's centennial goal of reaching "communities…not now reached by the Association." However, the bags of letters received by the Y.M.C.A. commending them on their association with "Sports College" also contained requests for publications. The publications cost money as did the secretarial services necessary to process all of that mail, respond to the letters and send out the literature. The Y.M.C.A. was not financially equipped to deal with the budget "Sports College" needed, which was obsolete within a matter of months and required a 50% increase for the second year. Nor were they mandated to hold any debts on their books. The National Council of Y.M.C.A.s praised "Sports College" for being "a fine example of a Dominion Broadcasting Corporation and a private agency co-operating in a fine service to boys and girls," but reluctantly announced that effective December 31, 1946, they would no longer bear the financial responsibility for "Sports College."

The CBC temporarily took over the funding of "Sports College" and considered making the arrangement permanent. Ernie Bushnell, Director of General Programs at the CBC since the end of 1944, advised his colleagues:

> The success of this program as I said before is astonishing and it is one program that I am sure we can cite with telling effect before a parliamentary committee.

Bushnell's right-hand man, Charles Jennings, lobbied for full CBC funding of "Sports College":

> It is important when we have an important series of this nature which can be of such great value to the corporation in its relations with so many groups throughout the country. ... Linked with this, of course, is the great prestige which we acquire with certain groups from such a program as well as the real value in the future when so many thousands of young boys across the country can view the CBC as bringing them this kind of radio.

The CBC Board of Directors, however, was reluctant to invest more than the estimated $100,000 per year of free air time that they had already committed to, and for eighteen months "Sports College" was in limbo. Some degree of private sponsorship had been an option from the beginning and with the runaway success of the program, serious proposals for large scale commercial sponsorship were received; however, Percival and the CBC rejected that option. In fact, Percival, the CBC and the Y.M.C.A. had already turned down a commercial sponsorship offer from a Canadian company which would have paid the Y.M.C.A. $50,000 per year and Percival $25,000 per year. Percival also rejected an offer from one of the big American networks which would have paid him at least $1,000 per week. Percival's refusal to accept the American offer as well as others that came later was, in part, a testament to his loyalty to Canada. But it also had to do with his unwillingness to relinquish creative control of "Sports College." It says a lot about the man and his "pugnacious individualism" that he turned down a minimum of $4,000.00 per month – the equivalent of well over $500,000 per year in 2013 – in order to carry out his mission on his own terms and in his own country.

The CBC paid Percival his $4,000 per year and underwrote the program's expenses during this time while corporate funding – as opposed to commercial sponsorship – was actively being sought. The Chairman of the CBC, Augustin Frigon, was fully behind this decision and was still considering making a long-term financial commitment to "Sports College." Frigon never had to make the decision. In the spring of 1948, a group of influential businessmen registered "Sports College" as a non-profit organization and guaranteed its financial viability. Percival gave up his offices, which had been relocated to the Central Y.M.C.A. building at 40 College Street West in 1947, and rented space on the second floor of a building at the northwest corner of Yonge and Wellesley Street. Perhaps there had been divine intervention. While the future of "Sports College" was still very much in doubt, Cardinal McGuigan, Archbishop of Toronto, wrote to Percival commending him on the program's "uplifting influence on our country" and concluded with, "While I wish you every success in this great work, I trust that you will receive whatever is required to maintain and develop your program."

By the summer of 1951, Percival had moved the offices of "Sports College" to 496 Church Street. He was also well-established as a track and field coach by this time and some of his athletes, notably Mary Lawrence, Paul Poce, Pat Galasso and Joe Taylor, contributed to "Sports College" as well as to the tabloid-style newspaper, the *"Sports College" Research Guide (SCRG)*, which Percival began publishing that year. The *SCRG* became a monthly publication in October 1952 and was renamed *Sports College News (SCN)* in the spring of 1955. Initially the *SCRG* was available for fifteen cents per copy and by subscription for one dollar per year; by 1955, it cost twenty-five cents and a subscription sold for two dollars for one year and an additional dollar for each subsequent year. The initial press run was an ambitious 40,000 copies, but Percival soon scaled this back to 25,000. This publication enabled Percival to explore issues of health and nutrition while also dispensing advice on coaching and other issues more directly aimed at adults. The first issue included no by-lines except on a small piece by another of Percival's athletes, George Lynch; however, in future issues, Joe Taylor was listed as editor; Dorothy Percival, under her maiden name Dorothy MacDonnell, was named women's editor and articles were attributed to Percival, as well as to his alter ego, Lou Allan, and to his brother, Alan.

Prior to Joe Taylor joining the team, Dorothy and Alan Percival were Lloyd's most important supporters and assistants. Alan Percival was a professional hockey player but also acted as Research Director of "Sports College." In the beginning he was on the air almost as much as his brother, but his contribution diminished as the years passed. Since she was content to stay behind the scenes, we will never know exactly how much Dorothy directly contributed to the development and production of all things that were "Sports College." She was a highly skilled typist – could knock off the "Sports College" scripts that Lloyd routinely finished on Saturday mornings, while he dressed to go to the studio – and typed all of his most important booklets and pamphlets. Furthermore, Dorothy was there from the beginning, working side-by-side with her husband when the core ideas were being formulated and there was not enough time or money to get everything done, and Percival never tired of telling people how much Dorothy's help and support meant to him over the years.

Joe Taylor began a twenty-four year relationship with Percival when he became an employee of "Sports College" soon after joining Percival's Toronto Track and Field Club in 1950. Unbeknownst to

Taylor, "Sports College" did not have the money to pay his salary and the first five hundred dollars he received from Percival had been borrowed from Taylor's father. Joe Taylor assisted with the "Sports College" scripts, quickly established his credentials as a writer and used the experience to gain a position with *British Press* (now part of *Associated Press*). He divided his time over the following decade between *British Press*, the editorial desk of the *Toronto Star* and the varied tasks that Percival expected him to carry out for "Sports College."

With the radio program established as one of the most successful in the history of Canadian broadcasting and the publishing arm pumping out booklets and pamphlets, Percival turned to film and television. Along with former CBC announcer, Joel Aldred, and his Fifeshire Films Motion Pictures Company, Percival began producing "Sports College" television pilots in 1952. Contrary to internal CBC memos, Aldred remembered the pilots being of high quality. In spite of this, Percival was never offered his own television program. This is a bit of a mystery. With his quick wit, warm presence and complete grasp of his subject, Percival was a natural for the new medium and was a regular guest on CBC television programs. Joel Aldred believed that it was his own well-publicized dispute with the CBC which caused the CBC executives to pass on the programs he and Percival offered them. If Aldred was correct, it would be the only time in Percival's life when he was held back by someone else's controversial image.

In spite of the fact that Ottawa's rejection of his proposals had pushed Percival into creating "Sports College," he never abandoned his conviction that the federal government should play a central role in the promotion of sport and fitness in Canada. When the creation of a *Royal Commission on National Development in the Arts, Letters and Sciences* was announced in 1949, Percival saw another opportunity to make his case before the government. The fact that the words "sport" and "fitness" were nowhere to be found in the Commission's mandate did not deter Percival who presented a brief titled "Cultural Values of Sports and Health and Fitness Activities in Canada."

In the opening paragraph he established the historical basis for including sport and fitness in government cultural policy:

> Physical fitness and prowess in sport have been
> integral elements with the arts, letters and sciences
> in the great historic civilizations to which our
> own Canadian way of life owes so much, obvious
> examples ancient and modern, being Athens and
> England.

The remainder of the brief is devoted to explaining how "good sportsmanship" is directly related to "good citizenship" and how "physical fitness through participation in sport" contributes to better education, national health and a decrease in juvenile delinquency. Percival also pointed out that there is something to be learned from America's modern example of successfully "developing character and leadership" through sport and stated, "It has been said that coaching is the highest form of teaching and that the coach is in better position to influence character than the professor."

"Sports College" was singled out as an organization that "would merit annual grants in aid from the federal government," but so too were the "Y.M.C.A., Church organizations, Scouts, C.Y.O., etc."

Specific objectives that Percival suggested included the creation of "special coaching schools," "Physical Education Laboratories" and "a national publicity and promotion drive designed to make Canadian people fitness conscious." Some variations on these themes appear in every brief Percival delivered to the government, both before and after 1949. They also bear a striking resemblance to initiatives that the Canadian government would finally embrace twenty to thirty years later: the Coaches Association of Canada (1970), ParticipAction (1972) and the first National Performance Centre (1980). It may be a bit of a stretch, but the "Top Secret – 2010" scientific research centres that were an important adjunct to Canada's

Own the Podium program for the Winter Olympics in Vancouver can also be traced back to Percival's sixty year old proposal.

In fact, this submission to the Royal Commission is the centerpiece of all Percival's public policy initiatives. It grew out of his simpler proposals to the federal government in 1936 and 1943 and is less complex than policy manuals he would produce in 1969 and 1970. However, within it, one finds the key elements of those later documents, and we see just how early Percival had successfully broken down and analyzed the problems facing sport and fitness in Canada and how he had devised modern solutions, some of which have only been fully implemented in the twenty-first century.

The final report, released by the Royal Commission in 1951 and popularly known as *The Massey Report* after the Chairman, Vincent Massey, includes no mention of sport and fitness. According to Robert Fulford, this document is "the most important official document in the history of Canadian culture." Yet, Fulford has charged that the "history-making report was not about culture but only one slice of it." Fulford was not thinking about sport and fitness when he made these comments decades after its release, but that was precisely what Percival was referring to when he informed people that he was extremely disappointed that the Massey Report had focused only on "high culture."

Few members of the sports community knew, or cared, about Percival's attempts to legitimize the status of fitness and sport within the Canadian cultural mosaic; however, he found a sympathetic ear in a young journalist named Douglas Fisher. Fisher was a fresh-faced graduate of the University of Toronto where he had studied under intellectual giants, Northrop Frye and Marshall McLuhan. He was also a competitive swimmer who listened to "Sports College" every Saturday and "had all of the books." Frye, editor of the *Canadian Forum*, was curious about this thing called "Sports College" and sent Fisher out to write an article about the institution and the man who ran it. Fisher's article praised "Sports College" for the effectiveness of its style and presentation and noted the progressive nature of its content, but Fisher was particularly intrigued by Percival's attempt to integrate the gentlemanly traditions of British sport with the egalitarian and individualistic attitude of the Americans – the balancing act Percival performed as he "attempted to straddle two different positions in what might be called his philosophy of sport." Such was the nature of Percival's public persona that he attracted attention from people like Northrop Frye and Douglas Fisher, people who were seeking a broader understanding of Canadian culture. Fisher's discourse on Percival appeared in the June 1953 issue of *Canadian Forum*, alongside essays titled "Capital Punishment," "Paris that Thinks," "The many faces of Censorship" and "Sir Flinders Petrie and the Royal Ontario Museum of Archaeology." The remaining pages were devoted to art, poetry, a short story and book, film and poetry reviews. This was not the company Percival was used to keeping, but he was definitely not out of place.

Hockey

THE SAME YEAR THAT *The Massey Report* was released, Percival published his most popular work. Although he wrote constantly, published articles, pamphlets and booklets on a wide range of subjects, *The Hockey Handbook* was the only full-length book Percival produced. It represented a quantum leap forward in hockey instruction not only because Percival produced the first detailed manual for understanding and coaching all aspects of the game, but also because he provided a fresh blueprint for teaching and playing hockey. He was unimpressed by the argument that Canadians played the best hockey in the world, that since the National Hockey League was the best of the best there was no reason for change. Percival knew that the game could be better and wrote *The Hockey Handbook* to help coaches make it better.

The Hockey Handbook covered the same basic material as *How to Play Better Hockey*. But with more than five times the content, Percival was able to include more detailed explanation and many additional drills for coaches to use. The text was still dense, with over five-hundred words per page, but included many diagrams as well as pictures of NHL players and action photos. The eight chapters: "Skating"; "Scoring Goals"; "Carrying the Puck"; "Offensive Strategy and Tactics"; "Defensive Strategy and Tactics"; "Goalkeeping"; "Practice Organization and Coaching Technique"; and "Training" included detailed instructions on every aspect of the game of hockey. The added research done through "Sports College" after 1944 and the time to develop specific drills for each facet of the game allowed Percival to produce a manual so complete that it had no rival for at least three decades.

One of the great merits of this book, and the main reason that it stood alone for so long, is Percival's insistence on breaking down and teaching the fundamentals of the game – building blocks for the hockey player which were deemed 'natural' skills and were therefore rarely taught. The greater the natural talent in the individual, the better the hockey player he would become. Or so it was assumed. There is some truth in this and it was certainly more relevant at that time, when Canadians developed their hockey skills through hours of shinny on the pond and the backyard rink. But Percival knew from his research that even marginal improvements in athletic ability, gained through scientifically devised training, would lead to improved performance.

The first chapter of *The Hockey Handbook* deals with skating, because skating is obviously the essence of hockey; however, prior to Percival, little was known about the technique of skating for the hockey player. As recently as 2002, when Alain Hache examined the biomechanics of skating for his book *The Physics of Hockey*, the only scientific research relevant to skating that he could find came from the sport of speed skating. Even though Percival had argued in 1951:

> There is just as much technical skill and training
> needed to skate well as there is to run, jump,
> forward pass, or throw a curve ball. There is no
> such thing as a born skater.

With the same kind of attitude, *The Hockey Handbook* approaches every aspect of the game of hockey and presents the reader with an easy means of understanding all that is essential and all that can be improved through specific drills and hard work.

The chapter devoted to goaltending is of special interest because the off-ice drills Percival devised were without precedence in hockey coaching. Furthermore, the drills using tennis balls to strengthen the hands and improve eye-hand co-ordination would have great historical significance. Of almost equal fascination is Percival's attempt to promote ambidextrous goaltending, which he declared "is likely to be one of the most important improvements in general goalkeeping practice to be made in the future." At this time, the goalie's 'catching glove' was not very different from the glove he used to hold his stick and Montreal goalie Bill Durnan was winning Vezina Trophies while switching his goal stick from hand to hand, depending on whether the opposition was attacking from the left wing or from the right. Soon after *The Hockey Handbook* was published, the goaltender's catching glove evolved into a true catching mitt and ambidextrous goaltending became a thing of the past. Still, this chapter exemplifies Percival's constant search for innovative ways to improve a sport that was heavily shrouded in tradition.

The final chapter, titled simply "Training," introduces a completely new physical, mental and dietary approach to the game of hockey. Percival discounted the prevailing wisdom that "the best way to get into shape for hockey is to play hockey," and presented a comprehensive guide to pre-season conditioning, regular season conditioning and off-ice training including: interval training, strength and flexibility work, an understanding of the role of lactic acid build-up in muscle fatigue and the resultant need for proper "cooling off," and the role of psychology in coaching. None of this was part of the North American hockey player's life in 1951, and the concepts were so radical that this book is worthy of study simply for its historical importance. The ideas are still so fresh, however, that it merits inclusion in the library of any modern day coach. At the end of the 1980s, highly respected Canadian goaltending coach Larry Sadler spearheaded a drive to produce a more up-to-date version of *The Hockey Handbook*. Experts from Hockey Canada were assigned to examine each chapter and asked to make recommendations on how to update and improve on Percival's work. The experts were "surprised at how much detailed technical information was in the book," and how little change was required. Although they modernized the book in terms of graphics and design and made improvements to the chapters on "Goaltending" and "Training," the editors of the

1992 revised edition left Percival's text virtually intact, acknowledging that it was still "the most technical book ever written on hockey."

The Hockey Handbook was a publishing success. In spite of its failure to find acceptance with professional coaches, the book found a home in the bedrooms of young hockey players all across Canada and in many a minor hockey coach's library. It had a significant impact on grassroots hockey development in Canada and was especially influential with university and college coaches in Canada and in the United States. In Europe and in Russia, *The Hockey Handbook* became the standard textbook for hockey coaches.

A great deal of *The Hockey Handbook* was written at the 'purple cottage' on a rock outcropping in Stoco Lake, near the town of Tweed, Ontario. Lloyd and Dorothy purchased the cottage in the late 1940's. On the rare weekends when Lloyd relaxed at the cottage with Dorothy and often with friends, he kept angling records worthy of a research scientist. In an August 1962 *Globe and Mail* column devoted to fishing, Percival reported that over a ten year period, he and Dorothy had caught forty-nine muskellunge in 756 hours of fishing including: twenty-five over twenty pounds, eleven over thirty pounds and two over forty pounds. Lloyd broke down the figures according to catches per month and hour of the day, recorded the weather conditions for each catch and the bait or lure that had been used. Dorothy caught her fair share of the larger fish and landed the biggest muskie reeled in at the 'purple cottage'. Lloyd sometimes made reference to this when he spoke to reporters about their close relationship and how, only because it was Dorothy, could he accept that someone else had caught the biggest fish.

The 1950-1951 Detroit Red Wings

At the beginning of the 1950-1951 hockey season, while awaiting publication of *The Hockey Handbook*, Percival offered his personal services as well as those of "Sports College" to any and all National Hockey League teams. Only the Detroit Red Wings expressed an interest – his home town Maple Leafs said they would allow him to do some tests on their junior team. As always, Percival expressed disbelief that the NHL as a whole failed to recognize the value of what he was offering. He should have been more surprised that even one team was willing to experiment with his programs. The NHL supported "Sports College" in the early days and, as long as Percival was simply advising young boys on physical fitness and helping prepare them to fulfill a dream of one day playing in the NHL, the league was supportive. As "Sports College" evolved and more and more of the advice on nutrition and exercise Percival dispensed each Saturday morning ran contrary to the traditional practice of NHL teams, support dissipated. This was especially noticeable in Toronto where the "Sports College" staff members were reduced to sneaking into Maple Leaf Gardens to conduct research.

The strained nature of Percival's relationship with the Maple Leafs was amply demonstrated in December 1951 when the bizarre controversy surrounding Eric Nestorenko became public knowledge. Nestorenko was big and strong, a proven goal scorer, and pegged to be the next superstar to wear a Toronto Maple Leaf uniform – Conn Smythe is said to have "bragged to the press" that Nestorenko would "one day make the hockey world forget about (Jean) Beliveau." Nestorenko was also one of the most interesting and individualistic hockey players of his generation. In order to get himself fit for his upcoming season with the Toronto Marlboro junior team, Nestorenko spent the summer of 1951 training with Percival's Toronto Track and Field Club. He returned to hockey in the fall, but he returned a convert to the Percival doctrines on fitness and nutrition. The most obvious change in Nestorenko was that he abstained from the traditional pre-game steak dinner in favour of yogurt and fruit. While Nestorenko was scoring and the team was winning, his unorthodox behaviour was tolerated. When he lost weight and stopped scoring, and the team went into a slump, manager Stafford Smythe blamed Percival's diet and ordered Nestorenko to fall into line. *The Globe and Mail* reported:

> Much to the chagrin of the Maple Leaf hockey
> organization in general, Nestorenko is a Lloyd
> Percival yogurt – grape – apple convert. And
> nothing the Marlboro management or his
> teammates can say has shaken the young star from
> his beliefs.

Percival responded through the press by arguing that Nestorenko
was not scoring because Smythe was forcing the young man to play
when he had a "heavy cold."

Nestorenko had to endure taunting from opposing players
(one of the more benevolent nicknames he was given was 'yogurt'),
occasional scorn from his own teammates and the abuse from the
Smythe family, but the young man was imbued with a great deal of
inner strength. He stuck to his beliefs, the other players eventually
accepted him for who he was and Maple Leaf management finally
left him alone. Nestorenko never blossomed into a superstar, and
the Maple Leafs eventually gave up on him. He did, however, enjoy
a long and distinguished NHL career with the Chicago Blackhawks
and managed to do it on his own terms. As well as having his name
inscribed on the Stanley Cup and playing in two NHL all-star
games, Nestorenko has the distinction of being one of the first
NHL players to attend university and certainly the only player ever
to have been enrolled in full-time studies during the hockey season.
The Blackhawks reluctantly accepted Nestorenko's demand that
he be allowed to miss practices and fly in only for games while he
attended the University of Western Ontario in the spring of 1956.
This arrangement would not have been possible had Nestorenko
not embraced Percival's off-ice health and fitness regimen.

Whether it was because they were more progressive in Detroit,
or simply that management wanted to steal something from under
the noses of their competitors in Toronto, the Detroit Red Wings
accepted Percival's offer and invited him to Detroit. Percival and his
staff arrived on December 4, 1950, and spent the weekend putting
the players through tests to determine their levels of strength, fitness

and hockey skills. On the following Wednesday, Percival and his staff joined the players on the train to Toronto, where the Red Wings had a game scheduled against the Maple Leafs. The seven and one half hour journey was spent conducting interviews with each of the Detroit players. The report Percival submitted, along with tables of test results for the individual Red Wing players, included a conclusion that, "when compared to other hockey players and teams evaluated, the Detroit club (had) by far the best all round balance and rating." Since Percival's findings on other NHL players had necessarily been done from some distance, this comparison to other teams was certainly flawed but it pleased Detroit General Manager, Jack Adams. Another comparison which came out of this study also made Adams very happy but proved to be a major stumbling-block in Percival's life-long struggle to gain acceptance from the inner-circles of the NHL.

On February 8, 1951, *The Detroit News* printed a story that led with "Detroit's Gordie Howe is the best right wing in hockey today, according to scientific tests that left Rocket Richard trailing a poor second." The story continued, "Tests conducted by Research Director (of "Sports College") Lloyd Percival over a 17 game comparison between the two players "scientifically" show Howe the master 16 to 1(categories)." Percival insisted that the research was undertaken on behalf of Paul Chandler of *The Detroit News* and pleaded, "I drew no conclusions from these figures. I merely supplied them." We can be certain, however, that Percival revelled in the publicity as did Adams and that the two of them were much more than innocent bystanders.

Dick Irvin Sr., coach of the Montreal Canadiens, was in Toronto for a game against the Maple Leafs when he was informed of the story on February 9. He was livid. Most of what he said was unprintable, but the newspapers could report that Irvin called Percival's comparison "the product of the brain of a child." In response to a reporter's enquiry as to the age of the child, Irvin said, "a three year old child." Irvin was not alone in his reaction to the story. The

Rocket was almost a god in Montreal. Members of the Montreal organization and their fans saw this as an affront to his honour and therefore to theirs. Even outside of Montreal, Percival's credibility was challenged. Richard was considered the greatest player in the league by virtually everyone who knew anything about hockey. Howe was good, but he was still young. To compare them at all was foolhardy; to pronounce Howe superior, and so dramatically so, was heresy. Howe's extraordinary career would eventually vindicate Percival. But Percival was never released from the purgatory to which NHL coaches and officials relegated him for daring to challenge their knowledge of the game. Sales of *The Hockey Handbook*, on the shelves less than a month, may have increased due to the publicity, but any slim possibility that people in and around the NHL would read the "pretentious effort" of the "bespectacled professor of a far-reaching empire known as "Sports College" surely disappeared.

The reports Percival submitted to the Red Wings were far more comprehensive and far-reaching than anything the Detroit brain trust could have expected. Individual player analyses were exhaustive – the report on Sid Abel "covered seven typewritten sheets and one recommendation suggested he spend 24 hours in bed after every 10 games." The team report, *First Report & Recommendations: Physical Evaluation, Detroit Red Wings Professional Hockey Team (World's Champions)* spans one hundred pages and dissects every facet in the preparation, development and performance of a hockey team. It had no precedent in the world of sport and remains today one of the most complete and innovative training manuals ever prepared for a hockey team. Percival promised that if the Detroit management and its players applied the program laid out for them "on a regular, well-organized basis," they would witness "a 25% improvement in fitness and mechanical ability in the first six to eight weeks and that the players would continue to improve throughout the year."

Today, it would be surprising to find an author devoting the first chapter in a hockey training manual to "Nutrition" (Part 1); in 1951, simply including this chapter anywhere in a manual on sport was audacious. Percival began his instructions to the Detroit players with sixteen pages on nutrition because, he wrote, "modern medical science now believes that nutrition is the single most important factor in the development and sustaining of top level physical fitness and mechanical skill."

Until not too many years ago, virtually all professional hockey players sat down on the afternoon of a hockey game and enjoyed a pre-game meal of steak and potatoes. This was considered so important that the parsimonious owners of the 1950s and 1960s paid for it. After the game, players would head for a bar and replenish their fluids by drinking beer. The continued reality of this practice can be seen in the list of "essentials" Team Canada took to Russia for the 1972 Summit Series – a list that began with three hundred steaks and large quantities of beer. Percival was the first to recognize the folly of this pre-game diet. He repeatedly advised NHL coaches and general managers that the benefits of the traditional pre-game meal were a myth and went so far as to say that filling up on steak and potatoes only hours before a hockey game would detract from optimal athletic performance. Percival's report states: "What is eaten **before** the game will affect the athlete's play and what is eaten **afterwards** will affect how he recovers from his efforts and gets ready for the next game." He suggested a large breakfast of six to eight oranges, eggs, dry toast and honey, yogurt, grapes, figs, bran muffins, coffee and clear tea, juice and six to eight Brewer's Yeast tablets. The pre-game meal, eaten two and a half to three and a half hours before the game (no more, no less), should include yogurt, grapes, juice, fruit, bran muffins, clear liquids sweetened with honey, and eggs (if not eaten at breakfast). The "jack-up" suggested one hour before or during the game was juice or tea with honey or dextrose. Percival advised saving the large steak for after the game when a player needs "protein to rebuild the tissue he had broken down." This was fifty years before scientific research led nutritionists to validate his position on protein replenishment. Percival explained that the player would also need a lot of "natural carbohydrates to replenish energy" and "alkaline foods to re-create his alkaline reserve." Few athletic trainers in the world understood any of these concepts, yet Percival was so sure of himself and so complete in his understanding of the lifestyle of the professional hockey player that he also made suggestions as to how the Red Wings should supply the players with appropriate foods on the trains they frequently boarded shortly after a hockey game.

Most of the following chapters in Percival's report for the Red Wings were equally incomprehensible to the typical hockey player and coach of that era, but almost all of them deal with concepts that have since become basic elements in the training of modern-day hockey players.

The chapter titled "Fatigue Recovery" (Part 2) explores the physical and mental benefits of improving the recovery rates of the Detroit players. The report states the players "will not only have a physical edge. ...knowing they will be able to recover quickly (they) will be much more likely to give their all when they are playing." Exercises designed to facilitate fatigue recovery are offered for players on the ice, sitting on the bench, in the dressing room between periods, immediately after the game and the morning after the game. All entail some sort of breathing, stretching, posture correction and replenishment of bodily fluids. Some suggestions, although theoretically sound, are absurd given the mindset of hockey players in the 1950s. Between periods of the hockey game, Percival requested that Gordie Howe, Ted Lindsey, Terry Sawchuck and the rest of the 1950 Stanley Cup Champion Red Wings lie down on their backs on the dressing room floor and extend their legs up against the wall. He told them that this was "a must" because "fatigue acids congregate in the legs" and "by getting them (the legs) up the job of the heart and lungs in purifying this blood is greatly eased." As impractical and unrealistic as this was, we now know that it was one of his most insightful instructions. Fitness experts, and society in general, have become more accepting of what yoga practitioners have known for centuries. Just as with breathing techniques and stretches that mirror those at the core of yoga practice, Percival's introduction of the Viparita Karani yoga asana, popularly known as the Restorative Inversion or Legs Up Against the Wall posture, and the importance he assigned to it was a stroke of genius.

Percival also advised the Red Wings to engage in "continued activity of some kind for 20 to 30 minutes" after the game in order to inhibit the accumulation of "fatigue acids" – now properly known as lactic acid. One suggestion was that players should "walk or jog slowly and easily around the dressing room or stationary in one spot" – stationary bicycles were yet to be invented. Again, it is not surprising that the Detroit players did not take to this; however, this idea of continued physical activity to alleviate the build-up of lactic acid has become the main focus of the "cool down" routine of every serious, modern-day athlete and a seemingly essential activity of every professional hockey player in the twenty-first century.

In the tests conducted for the chapter Percival dedicated to "Reflex and Reaction" (Part 3), only goaltender Terry Sawchuck distinguished himself. But it is interesting to note that the next highest potential scores were ascribed to future Hockey Hall of Fame inductees Gordie Howe, Red Kelly and Ted Lindsay. The drills laid out for the Red Wings were more elaborate than those found in *The Hockey Handbook*. As always with Percival, he began by stressing relaxation and included the standard drill he adapted to all sports. In this case, the skater was asked to intentionally tense all of his muscles then, on command, to relax completely. Percival believed that once a hockey player, or any other athlete, had a firm understanding of what tension felt like, he would be better able to free himself from it.

Terry Sawchuck received special attention in this section with five off-ice and six on-ice drills designed specifically to improve the reflexes and reactions of a goaltender. Included in the off-ice section is the "wall-ball drill" in which the goalie sits five feet from a wall with a tennis ball in each hand:

He then throws the ball in his left hand against the
wall and catches it as it comes back and then does
the same thing with the right hand. He continues
to alternate in this way, seeing how many times
he can throw the balls against the wall within ten
seconds. Then he should continue to do the same
thing throwing both balls at the same time.

In 1972, members of Team Canada would be in awe as they watched
Soviet goalie Vladislav Tretiak practice virtually the same drill. Team
Canada goalies Ken Dryden, Tony Esposito and Eddie Johnston
said that they had never heard of a goalie practicing anything
remotely close to this innovative off-ice training, in spite of the fact
that Percival had introduced it to the NHL more than twenty years
earlier.

Wayne Gretzky is our best example of a hockey player who could
"see the ice" better than anyone else, but has anyone ever heard of
a coach introducing drills to improve "Peripheral Vision" (Part 4)
and make players more like Gretzky? Percival outlined on-ice drills
as well as simple exercises that could be practiced at any time of
the day or night and included special drills to improve Sawchuck's
peripheral vision.

At this time, the health hazards of smoking had not been proven
conclusively and it was an ordinary part of life for a large portion of
the population. Many professional athletes still smoked and would
continue to do so for another twenty years. It was one of the things
that the Soviet coaches found so surprising about the Team Canada
players in 1972. Percival had always told athletes not to smoke and
the chapter, "Smoking" (Part 5), quotes extensively from a treatise
he published titled *Should Athletes Smoke?* which makes it abundantly clear that smoking is a health hazard and that "there are few
things that will cut down on his (the professional athlete's) efficiency,
shorten his career and be a detriment to his career than smoking."
Percival's detailed list of the deleterious effects of smoking goes
well beyond what you might expect to see, even from anti-smoking

lobbyists of that era, and refers to numerous scientific and "Sports College" studies. Percival offered "practical suggestions" to any player interested in quitting smoking and informed management that "it is impossible … to get their full money's worth from a man who smokes."

"Endurance" (Part 6), or the athlete's "ability to resist fatigue," was one of those prime areas where "good enough" was good enough for the NHL. By the standards of international athletes, the Red Wing players scored very low on the tests administered by the "Sports College" staff. Percival stated that he could dramatically improve those scores, and that the ability to perform at or near their peak would be a huge advantage to the Detroit team. We are reminded of the weary Canadian players in 1972 reporting that the Russian players "come at us in waves." Observers noted that there was no waxing and waning, as would be found in a Canadian hockey game, because the Russians wouldn't allow it. In the post-2006 "New NHL," this style of play has come to dominate, and only a team that has the ability to play this way for sixty minutes, game in and game out, has a chance of advancing through the playoffs and winning the Stanley Cup. Had Detroit fully embraced this part of Percival's report in 1951, hockey history would have changed dramatically.

Percival identified "Staleness" (Part 7) as a "mental condition that has physical symptoms." It is also called "burnout" and overwork is usually given as the cause. Percival, however, maintained that it is rarely the amount of work an athlete does that causes the problem. Rather, it is the food he or she eats and the variety of exercises and drills that make up his or her training routine. Staleness, he added, affects people in all walks of life where there is "a lack of variety in the work the person is doing." Percival's solution was an improved diet, a greater imagination from coaches in organizing practices and, in extreme cases, rest and a short-term, complete disassociation from hockey – an intervention that was unlikely to find favour with any NHL coach or general manager of that era or any other era for that matter.

The best example Percival could cite of how hard work would not "burnout" an athlete was on the ice every day in Detroit. Gordie Howe was the hardest working player on the Detroit team. Staleness or burnout was never a problem during his amazing thirty-three year professional career. During his first few years in Detroit, some sportswriters suggested that Adams and Ivan were "burning the kid out" by playing him more than thirty minutes per game (Howe sometimes got his rest by dropping back to defence rather than sitting on the bench). After concluding from his testing that "we've never looked at anyone like Howe," Percival informed the sportswriters that Howe was in no danger of "burning out" and, in fact, suggested that Detroit should take advantage of the tremendous physical and mental skills of the twenty-two year old and play him more. In a 1964 interview, Howe admitted that he did occasionally grow tired and that it was at those times that he found Percival's exercises "particularly valuable."

With "Learner Testing" (Part 8), Percival tackled an issue that was so far from the repertoire of any NHL coach that one wonders at the audacity, or perhaps the foolhardiness, of including it in this report. Learner testing referred to psychological research that was relatively new in 1951. In Percival's words, "people learn skills, develop knowledge and remember things in three basic ways – with their eyes, through the things they see; with their ears and the things they hear and by their body, by the things they do, the movements they make." Percival suggested that if coaches and players were given the means of understanding whether individual players learned best through visual, audio, or motor instruction, teams would be able to tailor instruction to the individual needs of each player, and players would be able to pay particular attention to the mode of learning that best suited them. Remembering that Percival learned his trade from coaching greats like Knute Rockne, who taught a respect for the individual needs of athletes back in the 1920s, Percival might be forgiven for thinking that he could introduce this radical concept to the NHL. But there were no Knute Rockne's in the NHL.

Percival also devoted chapters to "Flexibility" (Part 9) and "Mobility" (Part 10), prepared a wall chart of stretches for the Detroit dressing room and advised the players to do these exercises before practice, in their pre-game warm-up, between periods and after the game. He observed that many NHL players could only turn in one direction and asserted, "there is not one player on the team who could not develop a 10-25% skill, mobility, reaction or speed improvement." Gordie Howe was generally strongest in all areas that Percival tested, but even he was not perfect because, according to Percival, "even the greatest of athletes have weak spots." However, he argued, "even though there has not been a perfectly mobile athlete up until now there is no physiological reason why there could not be."

Some "Miscellaneous Factors" (Part 11) included in the report are arcane and even humorous, but others are prescient, not just as applied to hockey but to sport and society in general. For "Avoiding and Treating Colds" (Part 11 A), Percival suggested good nutrition, plenty of rest, 50,000 units of Vitamin A per day, cold showers to close the pores and the wearing of a hat. The "Use of Water" (Part 11 D) by athletes was just beginning to become controversial at this time. Most people still held to the belief that drinking water before, during or immediately following athletic endeavours would cause stomach cramps or worse. It is hard to believe today, but marathon runners routinely denied themselves any liquid replenishment for the duration of the event for fear of upsetting their stomachs. Percival was one of a small but growing fraternity that disputed this. Here he argued, "when the water content of the body is depleted through hard physical activity, it should be replenished." His advice falls short of our present day understanding of water intake requirements. But his suggestion that "the best rule for the athlete in regards to the water drinking problem is to drink water whenever he feels like drinking water" was certainly more accurate and more helpful than what most coaches were espousing at that time.

Regarding "Sex" (Part 11B), Percival wrote:

> Sexual release is actually beneficial to both the
> player's physical fitness level and his state of
> mind and emotional stability when it is properly
> scheduled and under ideal conditions.

Recognizing that individual needs differ and, as always, stressing the importance of proper nutrition, Percival suggested that "the detrimental effects of sex mainly come from the mind and the emotions, not the actual physical reaction." He advised that it is acceptable to have sex less than twenty-four hours before a game unless the player will worry about the effect it may have on his athletic performance – just as guilt over "an affair" or about masturbation would impede performance. It is the emotional conflict, not the act, which causes the problem according to Percival.

This was a remarkably modern attitude regarding a subject that was still very much "taboo" in sport and would remain so for many years, and it would have been interesting to see Jack Adams's face when he read that part of the report. The vast majority of sports people at that time worried about the physical and emotional effects of sex before a big game and sequestered their teams away from wives and girlfriends – a practice which continued for decades. Adams took this a step further and wished that his players would abstain from sex during the hockey season. In his biography of Gordie Howe, Roy MacSkimming has written: "Like Jack D. Ripper, the demented U.S. Air Force Officer in the movie, *Dr. Strangelove*, he (Adams) harboured a paranoia about a player being robbed of his 'precious bodily fluids.' "

Percival was one of the pioneers in sport psychology and it is disappointing that both *The Hockey Handbook* and his report to the Detroit Red Wings are weak in this area. The short section in the report on "Work Levels" (Part 11F) offers limited advice before concluding:

TECHNICAL SKILL IS IMPORTANT, OF
COURSE, BUT IT IS THE ABOVE FACTORS
(mental preparations) THAT FORM THE
PLAYER'S TALENTS INTO A MOULD
OF TOP LEVEL EFFICIENCY. ... THEY
CERTAINLY ARE THE SECRETS OF GREAT
PHYSICAL EFFORT AND GREAT PHYSICAL
CAPACITY

When Adams hired Percival, he surely did not anticipate such a tome, and the team did not incorporate all of Percival's suggestions. Therefore, it is difficult to assess the impact Percival had on the Red Wings and their success on the ice; however, the Detroit Red Wings of 1950 to 1955 rank with the greatest dynasties in NHL history and the 1951-1952 team, the one which was most impacted by Percival's modern techniques, was the best of the five – "possibly the greatest hockey club ever, at least over the course of a single season." Percival had nothing to do with assembling the talent on these teams, but many of his suggestions did find their way into the Tommy Ivan's practices, and Adams was quoted in 1964 as saying:

> Percival gave us a lot of valuable help and I recall
> that the smarter the hockey player, the more
> attention he paid to Percival. I'm talking about
> men like Howe, Kelly and Sawchuck – and it's no
> coincidence that those three are still in the NHL
> thirteen years later.

The end of the Red Wing dynasty coincided with the last vestiges of Percival's influence. In listing reasons for the decline in Detroit's fortunes, the trades made by Adams usually tops the list, but Adams blamed the new players and their unwillingness to accept Percival's unfamiliar training methods:

> After those big years some new younger players
> started to come along that just didn't seem
> interested in learning new ways to train for the

game. But as I said, the smart ones stayed with
Percival's system and stayed in the big time.

As a comprehensive program, Percival's detailed one hundred
page "Report" was doomed from the start. That program was
decades ahead of its time and may still be unmatched in the integrated and holistic approach it took to every aspect of the training,
conditioning and preparing of a hockey team. The failure to understand Percival's vision in its totality is unfortunate because the whole
was greater than the sum of its parts. The parts, however, were
each, in themselves, a distinct improvement on anything ever before
attempted in the NHL, and the fact that some of them found their
way into the training and coaching of these players is significant.

In 1964, Red Kelly stated:

> One of Percival's ideas that gave the Wings an
> edge over the other teams when we were breaking
> all records for consecutive league championships
> was his (Percival's) "sitting on the train" exercises.
> Other teams had to come off a long train trip
> and maybe have to go straight to the arena with
> cramped muscles. Percival showed us how to
> exercise while sitting down and that was a big help.

The Detroit players were given figs to eat. One day Adams appeared
in the dressing room with bunches of bananas, dropped them on
the training table and said, "eat these, they're full of potassium" and
Howe, along with some of the other players, chose poached eggs
over the traditional pre-game steak. Players also remember that the
team started to drink tea with honey while on the bench without
knowing why, and that the buffet on the train that Percival discussed
in the nutrition section of his training program was introduced without any explanation. There were individual players who knowingly
incorporated Percival's teachings into their approaches to the game;
others incorporated teachings without knowing that they came
from Percival, and some learned to see hockey in a different light.

As Percival so often stated, "inches make champions." The "inches" he provided helped make the Detroit Red Wings of the early 1950s the dominant team in the NHL and one of the best ever.

Percival's contribution was most immediate – and most controversial – in his work with Terry Sawchuck, who died tragically in 1970 at the age of 40 after a barroom dispute between him and New York Ranger teammate, Ron Stewart, spilled over into the front yard of their Long Island home. By this time, Sawchuck had earned a reputation as one of the most cantankerous of all professional athletes and as bad a practice goalie as ever donned an NHL jersey. He wasn't always that way. The late Max McNab, Hall of Fame player and executive who roomed with Sawchuck in the minors, remembered him as a "big, happy puppy dog." That's the Terry Sawchuck Percival began working with in 1950 and the hockey player Percival reported was:

> Good now and will probably become great anyway. But if he uses such side helps he will become greater sooner and get closer to his full potential than anyone has ever done. He has a magnificent body that if trained to peak skill will probably enable him to reach heights never before attained. This is a plain physiological fact.

In an April 12, 1952, segment of "Sports College" titled *Facts About the Terry Sawchuck Story*, Percival and Pat Galasso discussed the role of "Sports College" in Sawchuck's development over the preceding two seasons:

> Terry didn't seem to use his remarkable reflexes, coordination and agility in keeping goal. We found that the muscles in the back of Terry's legs were short and restricted his movement. Once he went to work on stretching these muscles he gradually began to improve. He has worked so hard on these drills that it would be pretty hard to find anyone whose muscles are more flexible than Terry's.

One of the keys to Sawchuck's success was the extreme crouch position he adopted and his ability to make acrobatic reactions out of and back into this stance. It is doubtful he would have been able to re-invent goaltending in this fashion had he not done the work required to increase flexibility.

Percival found it more difficult to convince Sawchuck that his agility and coordination would improve even more if he shed some of his 200 pounds. Neither was the Detroit management overly concerned about Sawchuck's weight until he reported to training camp in September 1951 weighing 219 pounds. Adams immediately ordered his goaltender to go on a diet designed by Percival. Ten weeks later, Sawchuck weighed 193 pounds. By seasons' end his weight had reached 170-175 pounds, the level at which it would remain for most of his career. In 1951-1952, Terry Sawchuck produced "possibly the single greatest season ever enjoyed by a goaltender." Unfortunately, at the same time that Sawchuck was losing weight, the ornery, standoffish part of his personality was taking over.

Percival's diet received a great deal of blame for Sawchuck's metamorphosis. Even his mother is said to have tied the change in her son's demeanour to the diet. But the exacerbation of Sawchuck's drinking problems has to be taken into consideration. Even in the minors Sawchuck had been known "to become cantankerous, when he was drinking." In Detroit, he started to hit the bars with a group that included a couple of Detroit Lions Football Club members who had earned a certain notoriety for their barroom antics, and the pattern continued to the sad ending of his career and his life. It didn't help that Adams became so distressed by Sawchuck's gaunt appearance when his weight at one point dipped to 160 pounds that, much to Percival's chagrin, he prescribed stout for the goaltender. To be fair, Sawchuck's drinking must be understood in the context of the times. A great many hockey players of that era drank heavily and little was said about it. Furthermore, Sawchuck played through a great deal of illness, pain and chronic injury throughout his career and often played his best hockey when he should not even have been on the ice. His truculence, his fragile psyche and his self-medication has been the subject of much conjecture. As *Globe and Mail* columnist, Dick Beddoes wrote:

> Psychologists probed the dark recesses of his
> psyche and found a man standing on the edge of
> an emotional abyss, harried by flying pucks and a
> persecution complex. There was always one sure
> liquid escape.

It is clear that a diet did not send Sawchuck on his downward spiral, but a diet and increased flexibility did help him become one of the greatest goaltenders of all-time. He maintained that reputation in spite of a rather dissolute lifestyle and an almost complete disregard for practice throughout the latter part of his career. Recent research suggests that Sawchuck's reputation is built almost exclusively upon those first five years in Detroit when he practiced what Percival preached. Imagine what might have been had Sawchuck continued to follow the training methods Percival taught him in those pivotal first few seasons.

Red Wing players who credit Percival with affecting their careers include Ted Lindsay, who learned proper eating habits from Percival and remembers Percival being on the ice introducing new drills to the players during training camp and at various times during the five year period. Lindsay was receptive to these new ideas because he was already "into sports medicine," and trained on his bicycle in the off-season, but Percival was the first to teach him about these things.

Red Kelly credits Percival for giving him an appreciation of proper nutrition, and says that "Percival was a hard man to forget. Even in summer you would remember something he had taught you and you would work on it."

It is ironic as well as instructive that out of all the hockey players Percival worked with, Gordie Howe was his best student even though Howe was the one hockey player who needed Percival least. Howe said that "Percival and I saw eye to eye from the beginning." They became friends. Percival visited the Howe household in Detroit, met Colleen and their three boys, and Howe visited the Percival home in Don Mills on a number of occasions. Howe is one of those rare athletes who have innate physical abilities as well as an intrinsic understanding of his sport. Howe told Eric Hutton of *Maclean's* magazine, "a lot of the things he (Percival) recommended I found I had been doing instinctively and I got a big kick out of Percival being able to tell me why I was doing them right." That is not to say that Howe did not learn anything new from Percival or that Percival's specific instructions regarding fitness and the understanding of the body did not contribute to the longevity of Howe's career. On Percival's advice, Howe changed his diet, did some running, took up cycling during the summer and worked harder than any of the Red Wings on the drills and exercises that Percival designed for the team. It is just that so many lesser hockey players could have gained so much more from listening to Percival the way Gordie Howe did.

Howe repeatedly helped Percival with "Sports College." He volunteered to be the subject of a couple of Percival's training manuals, was a guest on the radio show and, in 1963, participated, along with Terry Sawchuck, in the instructional film "How to Score More Goals," which Percival hoped would be used by minor hockey organizations in Canada to teach the basics of skating, passing and shooting. It was produced with the financial assistance of Quaker Oats, but still sold for $139.95. Advertised as "Gordie Howe and Lloyd Percival, the greatest coaching combination in modern hockey, right in your locker room," Percival seemed to have had little success marketing this film. Ironically, the Russians used the film to help them understand what made Canada's greatest hockey player so special, and this made Howe something of a celebrity in the Soviet Union. While in Moscow for the 1974 WHA/Russia hockey series, Howe was surprised to find how many people recognized him on the street and called him by name – until he learned of the popularity of the "Sports College" film.

International Hockey

It is not surprising that the Russians studied Gordie Howe from a film made by Percival. Unbeknownst to Canadians, Lloyd Percival was an important influence on the development of modern hockey in the Soviet Union and played a critical role in defining the differences between the way the game was played in the Soviet Union and European countries, and the way it was played in the NHL.

Prior to WWII, Russians were experts at the northern European sport of Bandy – or "Russky hokkei" – a cross between soccer and hockey played by eleven man teams on huge ice surfaces using a short, hooked stick and a round ball. "Canatsky hokkei" was barely known in the Soviet Union prior to 1947. When international politics dictated that the Soviet Union adopt Canadian hockey, Anatoly Tarasov was one of the people charged with teaching the Canadian game to the Russians and quickly emerged as the dominant hockey theoretician in his country. Tarasov didn't have to look far to find transplanted Canadian hockey. The Scandinavian countries had already integrated the traditions of bandy with aspects of the Canadian game, learned through contact with Canadians playing hockey in Britain, and Czechoslovakia played a distinctively Canadian style of hockey due to the influence of the man recognized as the "father of Czechoslovakian hockey," Mike Buckna, of Trail B.C. Tarasov, however, was dissuaded from looking outside of Russia by his mentor, Mikhail Davidovich Tovarovsky, who told Tarasov that he was "not mature enough to see foreign hockey." Tovarovsky instructed Tarasov, "first you need to invent, to make up your own things. And when you are able to firmly stand on your own two feet, you will go and see." It must also be remembered that this was Stalinist Russia and one could pay a high price for importing western ideas.

The late Canadian sportswriter, Jim Coleman, frequently related a story told to him by Lethbridge Maple Leaf hockey player, Stan Obodiac, who was of Ukrainian decent, spoke fluent Russian and sent regular dispatches back to the *Lethbridge Herald* while the Lethbridge team was in Europe for the 1951 World Hockey Championships. According to Coleman, Obodiac described a meeting with Tarasov at the World Hockey Championships in Paris in 1951, where Tarasov enquired about Canadian hockey instruction and Obodiac handed the Russian coach a copy of Percival's book, *How to Play Better Hockey*. Obodiac did not mention the meeting with Tarasov in any of his dispatches. He was a fervent anti-communist, and Coleman later wrote that Obodiac admitted to having given the book to Tarasov "impulsively" and "never forgave himself."

There is also no evidence that Tarasov was in Paris in 1951. In numerous interviews and writings for Russian audiences, he referred to the 1953 World Championships in Switzerland as his first exposure to international hockey. Throughout his lifetime, Tarasov was reluctant to publicly admit to any outside influence on the formation of his coaching philosophy, and he never wrote about Percival or any of his books; however, in his last book, *Tarasov* – published posthumously and only in the United States – Tarasov discussed the influence of Tovarovsky, and how Tovarovsky informed him in 1951 that he was ready to see international hockey firsthand, "even the Canadians." Tarasov described a trip to Sweden and how he followed the Lethbridge Maple Leafs from town to town, attending practices and watching each of the exhibition games the Canadians played as they prepared for the World Championships in Paris. The exchange of a hockey instruction book between a Canadian hockey player and a Russian hockey coach in Sweden in 1951 – an exchange which neither man liked to talk about – may sound improbable; however, Obodiac's ability to speak Russian and the unique nature of Percival's pocket-sized book lends credence to the claim that Percival's book was the first printed material on hockey instruction that Tarasov read.

Russian hockey experts, including respected journalist Seva Kukushkin, knew about Percival's influence on Tarasov and remember hearing the story of Obodiac and Percival's *How to Play Better Hockey* book. Kukushkin also remembers seeing the Russian translation of this small volume, and Stan Stiopkin, now a hockey coach in the United States, owned a copy while studying at the Russian Academy of Sport in the 1960s. In addition, there are stories told of a visiting Russian hockey coach holding up the Russian translation of Percival's booklet at The Fitness Institute in the 1960s and announcing "this is our Bible."

Establishing that Percival's influence on Russian hockey most likely began in 1951 confirms that his ideas on training for and playing hockey were a seminal influence on the early development of hockey in Russia. Ideas that were being ignored by Canadian hockey professionals enabled the Russians to adapt to our game so quickly that they defeated Canada in 1954 and won the first World Hockey Championships tournament that they entered. The fact that Tarasov was the dominant force in Russian hockey, at least until 1972, ensured that Percival was a major influence on the way hockey in the Soviet Union matured during the next two decades and why Percival has been called "the stepfather of Russian hockey."

Still reeling from the loss to the Russians in 1954, Canada sent a much better hockey team to the 1955 World Hockey Championships, a team that included re-instated professionals. Reporters from all of the major Canadian newspapers, none of whom had been in Stockholm the previous year, were dispatched to Krefeld, Czechoslovakia, and CBC television, still in its infancy, also signed on. For the first time, a film crew was sent overseas and, for the first time in twenty-four years, Foster Hewitt left his perch in the gondola high above the ice at Maple Leaf Gardens to do the play-by-play live from Krefeld. The record of Canada's convincing 5-0 victory over the Soviet Union was flown home and televised in Canada the following day.

One of those who watched the CBC broadcast was Lloyd Percival, who began studying every scrap of film footage of Russian hockey he could get his hands on. Percival would not have heard the story about Obodiac and Tarasov until many years had passed, but, later in 1955, he was aware that five hundred copies of *The Hockey Handbook* were being shipped from New York to Moscow and became even more curious about how hockey was developing in the Soviet Union. Percival also used his many contacts in Europe to access information and soon became Canada's foremost expert on international hockey.

In 1956, Percival wrote, "Just how are the Russians going about the development of hockey players?" He noted that they were applying the same scientific approach that they had brought so successfully to other sports and that coaches devoted 75% of their two hour practice time to "conditioning and drills" while in Canada, "conditioning is given short shrift" and Canadian players "learn to skate, shoot, shift and check by emulation." Percival also denounced the Canadian "philosophy that the body is the answer to all problems." No one else, inside or outside of the NHL at this time, saw the Russians as any kind of threat to the NHL and the Canadian game, but Percival warned:

> Our system was good enough as long as nobody
> else came up with a better one, with a method
> that had as high a potential in the ever-progressive
> development of greater skill and physical capacity.

And he made the seemingly ridiculous prediction that if Canadians failed to introduce:

> 'new and improved' training methods ... it will not
> be too long before Canada is no longer the home
> of the best hockey players in the world.

Percival also pointed out to Canadian hockey people who had been ignoring him for so long:

> There is nothing new and mysterious about the system the Russians are using to develop hockey players. The tricks and techniques they are using, plus a lot they haven't thought of yet, have been described and recommended in detail for some years in hockey publications available through "Sports College."

At the 1956 Olympics in Cortina, Italy, reinstated professionals were not allowed to compete and Canada lost to the Americans as well as to the Russians. The Russian invasion of Hungary led to a Canadian boycott of the 1957 World Hockey Championships in Moscow. When it came time to assemble a team for the 1958 World Hockey Championships, national pride was once again utmost in the minds of Canadian hockey officials and fans. The Whitby Dunlops were invited to represent Canada in Oslo, Norway. Their coach and general manager, Wren Blair, did everything he could think of to strengthen the Dunlops including bolstering his team with former professionals and employing the modern training techniques of Lloyd Percival.

Percival prepared a dry-land training program and introduced some on-ice drills. Blair recalled that "since the players took their mission to return the World Championship 'Trophy' to Canada very seriously, they paid great attention to Percival's program." He believed that they gained a better understanding of "how to take care of their bodies" through exercise and diet and learned "how to prepare themselves physically and mentally" to play the Russians. Team captain, Harry Sinden, remembers the special training program that Percival prepared for their time at sea. Jack McKenzie, a devotee of "Sports College" who had introduced Blair to Percival, led the onboard fitness sessions and credited Percival with "preventing seasickness on the voyage over." Whitby prevailed 4-2 over the Soviet Union in what has been called "one of the great hockey games of the decade." Mackenzie credited Percival with "making the win possible." When asked whether Percival's training made a difference in Oslo, Blair replied "all I know is that we won."

By the time of the 1960 Olympics, the European hockey teams were also becoming competitive with the club teams Canada sent abroad because they had also been reading *The Hockey Handbook*.

Swedish hockey historian, Krister Ericsson, lists *The Hockey Handbook* as one of only "three early hockey books in Sweden." The other two books were extremely limited in scope and offered Swedish coaches very little help in the development of modern training techniques. The late Arne Stromberg, one of the fathers of modern Swedish Hockey and coach of the Swedish National Team from 1960 to 1971, wrote in 1972:

> A good help to me was that I as early as 1953 got a copy of Lloyd Percival's HOCKEY HANDBOOK, which I read from cover to cover at least twice. My good friend and colleague Ake "The Professor" Lundstrom gave it to me. He was a fan of Canadian hockey since "childhood."

That the two most important coaches in the development of modern Swedish hockey learned about Canadian hockey through Lloyd Percival and *The Hockey Handbook* helps us understand why Swedish hockey developed as it did and how they were able to defeat Canada to win in the 1962 World Hockey Championships.

In Czechoslovakia, hockey had already built a strong foundation upon Mike Buckna's introduction of pre-WWII Canadian hockey. When Buckna returned to Canada for good in 1949, he left behind a void; *The Hockey Handbook* helped fill it. A translation was never published in Czechoslovakia, but the book was used by many Czech coaches including Ludek Bukac, who played for the national team during these years. He later spent seven years as National Team Coach (1980-1985 & 1994-1996) and served in the same capacity for four years in Germany and six years in Austria. Bukac was introduced to Percival's book by Professor Vanek. Vanek spoke glowingly to all of his students about *The Hockey Handbook* as did Professor Vladimir Kostka. Before retiring to academia, Kostka played for his country. He also coached the Czech National Team from 1963 to 1973 and was behind the bench for many of their greatest victories including the gold medal match against the Russians at the 1972 World Championships, only months before the Canada/Russia Series. Like Tarasov, Kostka was both a national coach and the most respected hockey theoretician in his country. After Tarasov wrote his hockey instruction books, Kostka wrote the most widely-read Czech training manuals; however, according to Ludek Bukac, "Kostka's books looked a lot like Tarasov's, just as Tarasov's looked a lot like Percival's."

Percival's seminal work also found an audience in Finland where Harri Lindblad, an ex-president of the Finnish Ice Hockey Federation, introduced the book somewhere between 1953 and 1955. It was partly translated and used in the biggest clubs. Aarne Honkavaara got hold of his copy of *The Hockey Handbook* and had it translated in its entirety prior to the 1957 season when he led his club team, the Tampere Ilves, to the Finnish Championship "without losing even one game, a feat that has never been duplicated by another team." That year Honkavaara also coached the Finnish National Team to a fourth place finish in the World Championships in Moscow. He writes that the book was "the first comprehensive coaching book that I got my hands on" and that he shared it with a number of other Finnish coaches. The following year, Canadian Joe Wurkuunen was named the first full-time national team coach, and he drew upon *The Hockey Handbook*.

The Finns were slower to become truly competitive in international hockey, but two Canadian coaches helped them bridge the gap in the 1960s. Derek Holmes is another "graduate" of Percival's Saturday "Sports College" broadcasts and has been a hockey globetrotter since the end of the 1950s – including a term as Technical Director of Hockey Canada from 1974-1980. While playing hockey in England in 1961, he was asked to coach the Finnish National

Team. Unaware that Percival's book was widely used in Finland, Holmes immediately wrote his mother requesting she send over his copy of *The Hockey Handbook*.

The most famous Canadian ever to coach in Finland was NHL veteran Carl Brewer. After the NHL had reluctantly allowed his reinstatement as an amateur, Brewer played for the Canadian National Team in the 1967 World Championships where he was named "Best Defenseman" in the tournament. Brewer then spent a year as playing coach of the Muskegon Mohawks of the International Hockey League before the Finnish Hockey Federation asked him to be the playing coach for the Helsinki IFK as well as for the National Team. Brewer had only one year of coaching experience with the minor league Mohawks, but he had discovered *The Hockey Handbook*, and he re-read it while coaching in Finland. Brewer is highly regarded in Finland for his technical contributions to their hockey program, but more for the attitude he introduced, which was based on Percival's doctrine of the "Happy Warrior."

The St. Michael's Major Junior 'A' Hockey Club

During the years Percival spent working with the Detroit Red Wings and immersing himself in international hockey, he was also busy close to home subjecting his theories to rigorous testing.

Prior to the 1950-1951 season, the St. Michael's College High School in Toronto hired Charlie Cerre, a star hockey player at St. Michael's in the 1920s, as head coach of the St. Michael's Majors of the Ontario Major Junior 'A' Hockey League. Cerre was a fan of the "Sports College" radio program and used his copy of *How to Play Better Hockey* while coaching in Sudbury. He arrived in Toronto just in time for the publication of *The Hockey Handbook* and read it cover to cover many times. The book wasn't enough for Cerre, so he arranged to meet with Percival. The two discovered that they were like-minded, and Percival took on the role of trainer for the hockey team, a position he also held on the football staff at St. Michael's while Cerre helped coach for one or two seasons.

Cerre was an innovative hockey coach who loved statistics and did in-depth analyses of games including detailed charts and graphs of player movements, and scoring opportunities. He may have been the first hockey coach to apply the plus/minus rating system so popular with coaches and statisticians today. Percival was the perfect ally for Cerre. He did game-by-game breakdowns of the St. Michael's players, recorded statistics on checking, shooting and passing, and gave Cerre detailed suggestions on how the team's play could be improved. This was in addition to the off-season, regular season and playoff training programs he developed as well as his standard recommendations on diet and nutrition. Percival applied the same scientific rigour to the training programs he developed for the St. Michael's football team.

Cerre was the coach; however, behind the scenes, Percival played an important role. The practice sessions he suggested to Cerre included detailed instructions on how the practices should be organized and implemented. He didn't simply outline drills, as he did for Tommy Ivan, but also sent Cerre detailed instructions on the "art" of coaching. One letter sent to Cerre prior to a game in March of 1952 runs four pages long and begins with:

> Here are a few of the things that I suggest you
> concentrate on before the game on Saturday.
> These are the things that when sold to your players
> will make possible levels of effort, attention and
> drive that would not otherwise be possible. The
> things dealt with are some of the all-important
> imponderables that make all the difference.

And it concludes with:

> Finally, I suggest that you go over these things as if
> you were giving a speech at an important banquet,
> read them aloud, try to memorize them. On your

ability to sell this stuff to the boys, depends its
success.

I know it will take a little effort and be a problem,
but don't forget: THE ONLY BATTLE THAT
COUNTS IS THE ONE WITH YOURSELF.

Future NHL star, Bill Dineen, who was in his last year at the
school when Cerre and Percival took over said, "it was amazing what
he (Percival) did for us. We all benefited from the cardiovascular
work." Dineen gave much of the credit for the team's run deep into
the playoffs that year to Percival and adds, "I never saw that kind of
training anywhere else that I played." Murray Costello, who went
on to play in the NHL before becoming Canada's senior international hockey administrator agrees that "no one else ever put me
through that kind of work. He taught us that we could do more than
we thought – mind over matter." Hockey Hall of Fame inductee,
Dick Duff "learned about fatigue recovery" and how to push himself harder. He credits his long NHL career, in part, to the work
ethic he learned from Percival because no coach ever demanded as
much of him. Fellow Maple Leaf and Hall of Fame member, Frank
Mahovlich, knew of Percival from listening to "Sports College" and
remembers well his personal introduction, which came at his first
dry-land training session with St. Michael's, where the fourteen
year old drove himself "until he was sick." No NHL coach would
put Mahovlich through dry-land training, let alone something this
intense, even though he played for some of the game's most successful coaches including Punch Imlach and Scotty Bowman.

Percival was able to do things for Cerre that he was denied
in Detroit. For example, he produced a seven-page "Hockey
Survey Analysis" of a playoff game between St. Michael's and St.
Catherine's on March 19, 1952, in which body checks for both
teams are recorded, categorized, counted according to location on
the ice and the level of success, and connected to scoring chances.

Shoot-ins and recovery rates are also totalled, positional play is analyzed, and passes are tabulated according to their locations, their success rate and the reasons for their success. Furthermore, shots at and on the goal are counted and the location from which they were directed is analyzed, and the time of puck possession inside the blueline is recorded for each team. Along with conclusions in each section, Percival presented Cerre with a summary of twelve "General" comments and recommendations for tactics and improved play for the next game in the series. This is the kind of detailed breakdown of a hockey game that today's NHL coaches depend upon but was unheard of at all levels of hockey at that time.

Percival's title was trainer. He was obviously much more to the St. Michael's hockey team, however. Percival was a fine athletic trainer, one of the very best in Canada, if not in North America. Percival's regular attendance as trainer at the St. Michael's football practices, often with his dogs in tow, resulted in an unusual footnote to his engagement at St. Michael's College High School. In 1953, a contest was held to find a nickname for the senior football team. The winning entry was the 'Kerry Blues'. According to several accounts, the name was inspired by Percival's two Kerry Blue Terriers, Curly and Rocky, along with Gary Schreider's dog of the same breed. Gary was a football star at St. Michael's and a member of Percival's 'Red Devils' Track and Field Club who went on to be an all-star in the Canadian Football League (CFL), a lawyer, an Ontario Supreme Court judge and co-founder of the CFL Players' Association.

Track and Field

The Toronto Red Devils Track Club

PERCIVAL'S INVOLVEMENT WITH TRACK AND FIELD was the direct result of his efforts to broaden the scope and effectiveness of his work at "Sports College." A key ingredient in the success of the radio program, and one of the main reasons that Percival was able to present Canadians with the most up-to-date and useful information on sport and sport training, was his insistence that he subject the training programs, athletic equipment and nutritional products promoted on "Sports College" to rigorous testing before giving his stamp of approval. Essential to this testing and research was his recruitment of young athletes to be part of what he called the "Sports College Testing Group."

Percival started with seven boys in 1946; by 1951, there were fifty boys and girls. While the group never grew much larger, Percival aspired to working with a Testing Group that would include 5,000 boys and girls from all across Canada. The members of the group played the dual role of research assistants and lab rats. They helped Percival test the effectiveness of exercises and nutritional supplements, aided in compiling the data he presented on "Sports College" and assisted with the research used to write his publications. Members of the "Sports College Testing Group" traveled to London, Ontario to meet Drs. Wilfrid and Evan Shute, the pioneers in Vitamin E research. A paper published by Percival in 1951 on the findings of a research study he had done with the Testing Group on Vitamin E and athletic performance supported the brothers' claims regarding the miraculous powers of vitamin E, which were very controversial at that time.

Percival and his boys also visited Dr. Thomas K. Cureton whose Physical Education Laboratory at the University of Illinois was leading the way in physiological research in North America. Percival and Dr. Cureton corresponded regularly and shared with each other all of their findings. On one visit, the boys were subjected to a number of tests and Murray Gaziuk managed to get himself into the Guinness Book of Records by doing 2,228 consecutive deep knee bends; however, the "Sports College Testing Group" is best remembered as the heart of the most successful club in the history of Canadian track and field and one of the most dominant clubs in the history of all Canadian sport: The Toronto Red Devils Track and Field Club.

Of all of the athletes Percival would work with throughout his career, only the track and field competitors became part of a club, formally sponsored and coached by Percival. In 1951, he listed the reasons that he chose to devote so much of his time and energy in coaching track and field:

- This sport is exceedingly measurable and offers an ideal medium for testing and measuring the results of training, nutrition and so on.

- Progress and performance could be accurately gauged due to factors of times, distances and so on.

- There was a great need for the improvement of track and field standards in Canada.

- Something needed to be done to raise the threshold of ambition of the track and field athlete in this country. He needed to be shown that much better performances were possible.

While this scientific rationale is convincing and consistent with Percival's endeavours over the years, fate and circumstance may have been just as significant. At a cross-country meet in the spring of 1946,

Percival met George Lynch, a student at Lawrence Park Collegiate in North Toronto. After finishing eighth, in spite of having never previously run a race, Lynch asked Percival to personally supervise his "Sports College" training program. Percival agreed. One day, Lynch brought along a friend and it wasn't long before there was a group of very talented athletes from Toronto and area high schools training under Percival and forming the core of the "Sports College Testing Group."

Through the vast network of contacts he had established with his letter writing campaign of the 1930s, Percival was able to access the latest training methods being developed in Europe. The training programs he set for these young men proved to be so superior to the outmoded techniques employed by other coaches in southern Ontario that within a few months, Percival had turned his young athletes into the best young runners, jumpers and throwers in Toronto. After Lynch, Bruce Rawlinson and Kim Kimbark won their events and led a contingent of Toronto athletes to a fourth-place finish in the Junior Olympics, a city-versus-city Olympic-style competition organized by a Cleveland, Ohio, radio station in August 1946, *The Globe and Mail* reported: "Without fuss or fanfare Lloyd Percival is doing a commendable job of building a colony of track and field stars under the Sports College banner."

In 1947, the numbers swelled even more as word spread that Lloyd Percival, the "Head Coach of Sports College," had formed a track club. Percival formalized his commitment to the athletes with the formation of the North Toronto Track and Field Club (NTTFC). He nicknamed them the Red Devils, designed a distinctive logo and dressed them in bright red shorts, tops and track suits. The original core group was part of the club but retained its status as the "Sports College Testing Group," and its members sometimes wore a royal blue uniform with a "Sports College" crest. In time they were joined by other premiere athletes who were willing to put in the extra time required to participate in Percival's research studies, and the Testing Group became a kind of elite squad within the NTTFC.

The NTTFC infused life into a moribund track and field scene in southern Ontario. The best of the half dozen existing clubs was the West End Y.M.C.A. group coached by Hec Phillips. Paul Poce, the future Toronto Olympic Club founder and Canadian National coach, joined Phillips' club in 1946 and remembers, "just 5 or 6 guys using Cromwell's book." Cromwell was Dean Cromwell, the USC coach who had instructed Percival in track and field coaching and who had offered him a job in the 1930s.

The most ambitious and best athletes began leaving the other clubs and coaches to train under Percival. The defections sparked resentment. When mixed with Percival's impatience for coaches who didn't understand what he was doing and his penchant for self-promotion, conflict was inevitable. Percival was called "a parasite who lives off the labour of other track and field coaches." When Robert Fulford surveyed the scene as a reporter in 1950, he saw that "his (Percival's) status with 70 to 80% of the track coaches and high school teachers was negative. Sometimes they didn't even mention his name. You just knew who they were talking about when they said 'there was one coach who was burning people out'." According to Fulford, Percival wasn't just ahead of his time: "He was speaking a different language."

Joe Taylor left the West End Y.M.C.A. group in 1949 to join the NTTFC. He was followed by Poce in 1950, and, together, they gained firsthand knowledge of what made Percival's track club so different. Besides the commitment to train five or six days a week instead of the three they had been used to, Percival's workouts were much more intense and varied. After forty to fifty minutes of stretching, there was approximately one hour of training which changed constantly. One day they might leapfrog for almost an hour; Don Aitken remembers one workout where he and fellow middle distance runner Rich Ferguson began the session lined up on opposite sides of the running track. Their workout would not end until one caught the other, a game that might take more than one hour. Most sessions were more conventional, but the point was for each workout to be interesting as well as demanding. On occasion, Percival brought out a phonograph and played jazz records to keep the sessions relaxed. Sometimes the boys left the track to run hill repeats up steep Rosedale Valley Road or to run cross-country while wearing winter boots.

The most important of Percival's initial innovations to track and field training in Canada was the introduction of *fartlek* and interval training. *Fartlek*, a Swedish word that loosely translates as "speed play," involves bursts of speed and powerful surges over various distances and varying terrain. It was born in Sweden in the early part of the twentieth century and was the major reason that Swedish and Finnish distance runners dominated world distance running into the 1940s. *Fartlek* training moved to the track in the form of interval training when a few coaches began preaching that repetitions of shorter distances at a faster pace, with rest in between each, were a more effective method of training than running the same total distance at a slower constant pace. The birthdate of the modern era of distance running has been set around 1950 because Roger Bannister was introduced to *fartlek* in 1949 and began serious interval training in 1950; John Landy closed in on the four-minute mile mark when he began running a demanding regimen of intervals on the track in 1952, and the towering figure in American distance running, Bill Bowerman, began experimenting with interval training at the University of Oregon between 1950 and 1952. However, by 1947, Lloyd Percival had already incorporated these most modern aspects of track and field training into the daily routines of a group of Toronto schoolboys.

Percival's innovations in track and field training did not stop there. He introduced these young men to weight training; developed stretching regimens specific to the individual needs of their events and of their bodies – some of which were learned from a ballet instructor; took them to Archie Campbell, trainer for the Toronto

Maple Leaf Hockey team, for massage and athletic treatment; sent them to see a homeopathic doctor for more serious problems; and put them on special diets that were high in protein and low in sugar.

The diet that Percival designed for the Red Devils was particularly innovative and similar to the one he designed for the Detroit Red Wings; however, due to their regular contact and the age of his track and field athletes, Percival was much more successful in making the diet a part of the boys' daily routine. It included whole grain cereals and breads, vitamin E and B complex supplements, and various foods that he considered crucial to athletic development, including dried figs because he knew they were high in iron and alkalinity, large quantities of oranges for their vitamin C and yogurt. To the contemporary reader, this may seem rather ordinary advice. But Percival's conviction that dietary changes could have a major influence on athletic performance was shared by only a few international sports authorities of that era and was virtually unknown in Canadian homes where large quantities of white bread were consumed, vitamin supplements were extremely controversial, figs were considered exotic, oranges were seasonal and yogurt was a foreign word.

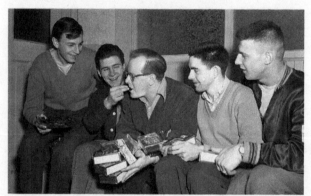

Lloyd Percival (centre) with members of the Sports College Testing Group: (left to right) Unknown, George Lynch, Lloyd Percival, Art Cowie and Murray Gaziuk, promoting the health benefits of 'Blue Ribbon' figs in 1949.

One source suggests that Percival became interested in yogurt after witnessing the strength of the Bulgarians at the 1948 Olympics; that he came home with the idea that it was due to the yogurt they ate and, after his typically exhaustive research, concluded that his athletes could derive many benefits from including a minimum of one pint – but preferably one quart – of yogurt per day in their diets. While this is consistent with Percival's history, he later wrote that it was an article in the *Canadian Medical Journal* that inspired him to initiate an eighteen-month study of the legendary "preventative" and "therapeutic" powers attributed to yogurt by the people of the Caucasian mountain area. Either way, Percival's adoption of yogurt as a "wonder food" was years ahead of nutrition experts and decades ahead of mainstream Canadian society. It was a testament to his curiosity, his intuition and his scientific rigour – not to mention his determination. Because yogurt was not available anywhere near Toronto, Percival and club members first travelled to La Trappe, Quebec, to obtain the culture. Soon he arranged to have The Roselle Institute in La Trappe deliver a monthly supply of the culture to the athletes' homes. The mothers of the NTTFC athletes were then responsible for making the large quantity of yogurt Percival prescribed. Eventually, Percival convinced a couple of Toronto health food stores – MacMillan's in Yorkville and Hooper's at Church and Bloor – to stock the yogurt culture.

Percival's advanced, holistic training model for track and field was firmly established by 1947 when most coaches in Canada were just learning how to use a stopwatch, and this is what Robert Fulford meant when he asserted that Percival "was speaking a different language."

Percival's greatest challenge was to find suitable competition for his young athletes at a time when there were only a few meets in Ontario organized for high school and university students. He began working behind the scenes. In 1947, the Gladstone Athletic Club hosted a Marathon Championship in East York that, for the first time, included a few junior events in its limited track schedule.

NTTFC runners dominated these events. In the fall, Gladstone was the host for the Canadian Cross Country Championships which also, for the first time, included a junior race. The race was won by George Lynch of NTTFC. The biggest step forward for track and field in Ontario that year came with the staging of the first annual Ontario Junior Track and Field Championships held at Varsity Stadium on June 28. Percival spearheaded this meet in which three hundred and twenty-five young athletes took part. NTTFC, in its first year of operation, won the team competition over the Hamilton Athletic Club, which had been around for more than a half a century. Percival arranged for private sponsorship and took seventeen of the best athletes from the meet out west to compete in the National Championships in Vancouver.

In February 1948, Percival took eight of the NTTFC boys to New York's Madison Square Garden for the National Amateur Athletic Union (NAAU) Indoor Championships for schoolboys. This would be the first of seven annual visits to this prestigious track and field meet for Percival's boys. In spite of top-level American competition and second-class treatment afforded the Canadians on their first visit, the Ontario schoolboys came home with six medals including Gordon Naight's gold in the 600 yard run. The Toronto newspapers heralded the boys' success. Percival was pleased with how far his young athletes had come but was under no illusions as to how they would fare against the best in the world. Since the Berlin Olympics in 1936, 1948 was the first year when athletes from around the world would come together. Track and field officials from all across the country were looking forward to how Canadian athletes would fare. Percival, as usual, had other ideas.

Percival's first couple of years in Ontario track and field and his travels across Canada with the Ontario athletes the previous summer inspired him to declare, "to me the first and foremost consideration is for the welfare of the competitor. Amateur officials in the main care only for the meet." Sports historian, Bruce Kidd, agrees with Percival's assessment of amateur sports officials from this era: "For many volunteers, the formal meetings, the elaborate public functions, and the endless lobbying and log-rolling behind the scenes took on a greater importance than the provision of opportunity for sports." The amateur sports officials in Canada contributed many hours of unpaid labour. Percival and other critics of the antiquated Amateur Athletic Union (AAU), the organization that governed sports bodies in Canada, were quick to recognize and even praise this contribution to amateur sport, but Percival "refused to accept mediocrity" and mediocrity was the currency of the AAU officials.

The AAU officials, or "badgers" as their critics preferred to call them, cherished the few benefits that accrued from their long hours of work. One benefit was the power they wielded. Any new ideas, such as those promoted by Percival, threatened that power. Another major benefit was travel and its incumbent perks, and the best trip of all was to the Olympics. When Percival told officials that sending a Canadian track and field team to London was "ridiculous," he threatened their first paid summer vacation in twelve years. Percival argued that Canadian track and field athletes were not ready to take on the rest of the world and, instead of picking a team at the last minute and dumping them into the middle of a track meet for which they were ill-prepared, it would be better, he argued, to "spend the money developing kids for the next Olympics, and the next." Andy Lyttle of the *Toronto Star* echoed Percival's sentiments: "Unlike other countries which gather material over long periods and train it with resounding accompanying trumpets, our method is hit or miss and devil take the hindmost badger at boatside." It is ironic that Percival had a paid trip to London, courtesy of the CBC. He proved to be a worthy student of Ted Husing and was equally adept as both a colour analyst and a play-by-play announcer. He was heard nightly in the Olympic summary which was broadcast over the national CBC network.

The 1948 Canadian Olympic track and field team proved to be woefully weak. The bronze medal won by the Women's 4×100 relay team salvaged a modicum of pride, but youth, a lack of international experience and limited exposure to modern training techniques left the Canadians up the track in almost every event as Percival had anticipated. He had also anticipated the behaviour of some of the badgers in London; however, the degree to which their antics affected the performance of the athletes inspired Percival to publicly lament that he was "ashamed to admit that he was a Canadian." Percival made this declaration after he learned that sprinter Jack Parry of London, Ontario, had injured himself in an unsupervised workout – unsupervised because the coach was "in London having tea." When the *Toronto Star* reported Percival's scathing commentary on the Canadian track and field coaches and officials in London, his already difficult relationship with Canadian track and field professionals became a canker that would fester for years.

After the 1948 Olympics, Percival also took to task the Canadian Olympic Association (COA) and the British Empire and Commonwealth Games Committee (BECGC) for failing to keep pace with the rest of the world thereby establishing himself as the black sheep of all Canadian amateur sport. Percival, however, could never be accused of throwing darts and walking away. In the aftermath of the 1948 Olympic disappointment, Percival "drew up a national sports development plan designed to raise standards of competition to contending levels in all sports." It was laid out in seven steps:

1. Talent identification, registration and tracking of developing athletes, so that "the controlling body, at a minute's notice, would be able to check just what material we have available for international competition."

2. Analysis of how and why some areas produce better athletes and correcting the inequalities through improved coaching.

3. A sport by sport analysis to help concentrate more on core sports such as hockey, track and field and skating until a larger "reservoir of talent has been established" in "Olympic fringe sports."

4. Identify and notify athletes considered "future representatives of Canada" and to instill in them "a definite desire to compete on behalf of their country" (something Percival claimed his research had proven was lacking.)

5. For the COA to concentrate on supplying coaching and technical support to these athletes.

6. Once each year identified athletes be brought together for training and development as well as progress assessment.

7. Every effort would be made by the COA and the other organizations participating in the program, to further publicize amateur sport, develop interest in all international competitions, and awaken a desire on the athletes' part to support and participate in those competitions.

The COA, BECGC and the AAU all received copies of this plan. Percival later stated: "At best, I merely got polite rejections."

The more inquiring sports journalists and editors saw Percival as a breath of fresh air – a kind of Robin Hood figure. It didn't matter that he was an unapologetic self-promoter, or that, like McLuhan, he sometimes courted controversy just for the sake of controversy; Percival was always well-informed and entertaining. When he poked holes in the establishment, it was obvious that he was releasing old, dead air. One sportswriter who used Percival in his continued assault on the amateur sport establishment in Canada was Andy Lytle of the *Toronto Star*, who wrote of Percival:

> Single-handed, he seems to do more for track-wise young Canada than the entire AAU set-up. …Wonder why they don't get behind Lloyd who long ago proved that he is an organizing genius as well as a practical theoretician. …Could there be a lurking green-eyed monster in the cinders?

And Bobbi Rosenfeld of the *Globe and Mail*, Canada's female Athlete of the Half-Century and one of 'the matchless six', the women's team that dominated the 1928 Olympic Games in Amsterdam, also deplored the lack of preparation that had doomed the Canadian athletes in 1948. In June 1950, Rosenfeld challenged the Canadian Olympic Committee to use the $14,000 that they had left over from the 1948 Olympics to hire Percival.

In 1949, a second successful foray to the NAAU Junior Nationals in New York yielded one first, two third and two fourth place finishes. Later that year the NTTFC easily won its third straight provincial Junior Championships. Percival began planning another trip to the NAAU championships at Madison Square Garden in 1950. Some months before the meet, Percival informed middle-distance runner, Charles 'Chuck' Tobias, that he would be entered in the mile run. Tobias knew that he would be competing against top American schoolboys whose times were superior to his own, but Percival assured him, "Don't worry, I have a plan." Throughout the winter, Tobias ran repeats of 600 to 1300 yards with the consistent aim of going out as fast as he could and then holding on. When they traveled to the NAAU meet in February, the race plan was set – run it like a training session. Since more than thirty runners were squeezed onto the track for each heat, Tobias was fortunate to draw a low number and ran from the front row. Because of the size of the field, and the difficulty in coming from far back, the best runners were forced to adopt Tobias's suicidal pace. None of them had trained as he had, and Tobias finished the race twenty-five yards ahead of his nearest competitor. The time was not great, but the strategy had gained Tobias the victory, caught the attention of the American coaches and eventually led to a track and field scholarship at USC.

For two years, Percival had been attempting to bring international, indoor track and field competition back to Toronto for the first time since before WWII. Having failed to find a company or an organization willing to put up the $5,000 required for a removable track to replace the one built for Maple Leaf Gardens that had been used as firewood during WWII, Percival settled for the hard concrete floor and cramped quarters of the Armouries at Toronto's Fort

York. On March 3rd and 4th of 1950, athletes from Canada and the United States competed in the first annual Eastern Canadian Indoor Track and Field Championships sponsored by "Sports College" and The Second Armoured Division. The NTTFC athletes performed well against the world-class American athletes who competed, but 'Reverend' Bob Richards was the star of the meet. He failed in his bid to break the Canadian record in the pole vault, but Richard's participation helped draw 3,000 people on the first night alone.

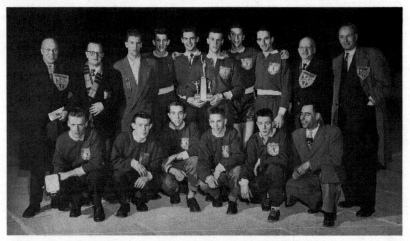

The North Toronto Track and Field Club around 1950.
Back row, left to right: unknown (1), Lloyd Percival, Norm Williams, Jack McRoberts, Don Ross, Murray Gaziuk, Gord Haight, Joe Taylor, unknown (2) and unknown (3)
Front row: Rich Ferguson, unknown (4), Peter Sutton, Don Aitken, unknown (5) and unkown (6)

In July 1950, at Toronto's Pantry Park, Percival organized, and the NTTFC hosted and dominated the first Canadian National Junior Track and Field Championships. Later that summer, pole-vaulter Ron Miller of the NTTFC finished sixth at the 1950 British Empire and Commonwealth Games in New Zealand – the Canadian team finished a distant, and disappointing, fourth in the medal count. Percival responded by putting together a National Sports Development Plan and submitting it to the AAU, the COA and the British and Commonwealth Games Committee (BECGC). He argued that Canada would have to start right away if it was to make a better showing when it hosted the 1954 BECG in Vancouver. AAU, COA and BECG officials were all quoted as saying that they supported Percival's proposals and would table them with their organizations.

By this time, the NTTFC Red Devils had left their North Toronto home and become the Toronto Red Devils Track and Field Club (TTFC). Club members now came from all over the Greater Toronto area – a couple of boys even commuted from Hamilton – yet the club had no single, established training base. Unable to acquire permits or perhaps too impatient to submit to all of the red tape required, Percival moved his club frequently to any available track that was accessible by public transit. Pantry Park, in The Beach neighbourhood of east-end Toronto, and Rosedale Park, where Percival had played cricket as a youth, were regular training sites; so, too, were Humberside Collegiate, Lawrence Park Collegiate and, in winter, the University of Toronto's Hart House and the RCAF station on Avenue Road.

One of the boys who joined at this time was John 'Jack' McRoberts. The TTFC was second choice for McRoberts because he lived in the east end of Toronto near the home of the Fred Foot's East York Track Club (EYTC). McRoberts' house backed onto the East York boundary but was not actually in East York, so Foot denied him membership in the EYTC. This was typical of the narrow parochialism endemic of coaches and officials in the Canadian AAU. While Percival was doing whatever he could and going wherever he had to in order to best serve the athletes, all too often other coaches settled with serving the rulebook and the status quo. McRoberts shakes his head at the memory but adds, "It was the best thing that ever happened to me."

Percival did not accept every boy who asked to join the TTFC. First he wanted to know about their family and their aspirations, but the only thing that really mattered was how they responded to tests of courage and desire. Even Rich Ferguson, who set a slew of Canadian junior records, was the 1953 NCAA two-mile champion and an All- American at Iowa and finished third behind Bannister and Landy in the 1954 "Miracle Mile," was considered by Percival to have no special physical attributes when he joined the club. While Ferguson benefited from the same advanced training, as did all of the TTFC athletes, Percival attributed his ultimate success to "his own excellent attitude, and success of the emphasis placed on personality and character development." Don Aitken followed Rich Ferguson from Leaside High School to a TTFC tryout. He was even less of a "natural" than Ferguson, but he gave everything he had and struggled to complete the tough initial workout Percival set for him. After the tryout, Percival took him on with the caveat, "you don't have the natural physique – you'll have to work harder." A few years later, Aitken followed Ferguson again – this time with a track and field scholarship to the University of Indiana.

The young men and women who joined the TTFC came from diverse socio-economic backgrounds. Bob Bazos' family owned Bell's Dairy which later became the Becker's Milk Company. They offered to pay for Bazos trip to Helsinki in 1952 after he failed to make the qualifying standard. Other athletes came from families wealthy enough to contribute to the expenses of the club which certainly could not have been covered by the $5.00 per year ($2.50 for those under 13) that Percival collected to pay for AAU memberships, meet entry fees, club uniforms and travel expenses. Some, however, like Ron Miller whose father died when he was two years old and who considered Percival a surrogate father, remembered Percival paying out of his own pocket to purchase track spikes for those who could not afford them. In fact, Murray Gaziuk believed his Ukrainian immigrant parents never paid one cent to the track club. If an athlete passed one of Percival's simple tests of character, he gave them everything he had and was almost always rewarded by the qualities that developed in the young men and women.

One young man whose growth both as an athlete and as a person had deeply impressed Percival was at the centre of the only truly tragic event in Percival's controversial career. On March 23, 1951, Percival accidentally shot and killed seventeen year old University of Toronto Schools student and reigning Canadian Junior Cross-Country Champion, John Vamplew, with a starter pistol. It happened at Pantry Park. Vamplew was sitting in the first row of the bleachers when Percival came over to "give him a pep talk." Percival put his left arm around the boy's shoulder; his right leg was on the bench beside the boy, his right hand loosely holding a starter pistol, rested on his right knee near Vamplew's chest. Percival remembered that they were talking about the Olympics when Vamplew suddenly jumped up and hit Percival's right arm. The gun pushed into the boy's chest and the trigger depressed. After the shot, Vamplew jumped off of the bench and ran, with Percival yelling after him, "Are you alright? Did you get a burn?" before Vamplew collapsed into the arms of two runners on the opposite side of the track. According to the autopsy findings of Chief Coroner, Dr. Smirie Lawson, the boy died "almost instantaneously," his death caused by "concussion caused from gasses of the exploded shell that tore through the chest and ruptured the muscles of the heart." Contrary to the Coroner's report, the boys remembered a thirty to forty minute wait for an ambulance, and Vamplew still alive when he left for the hospital. He was pronounced dead upon arrival.

Today, an autopsy might reveal some sort of heart anomaly in the young man, but today the ambulance would also arrive sooner and in time to perhaps save him. According to Dr. Lawson, John Vamplew's "death was one of the rarest accidents he had encountered in 20 years as a coroner" and no one was responsible. Furthermore, it was concluded that the starter pistols routinely used at athletic events were "very dangerous" and "could kill from six inches away." This was unknown to sports people in North America who were actually using ordinary pistols loaded with blanks because true starter pistols were manufactured in Germany and cartridges had been unavailable since WWII. The coroner recommended using cap pistols as a safer alternative. Although cleared of any wrongdoing, Percival was understandably devastated. He said that John was "the kind of kid great ones come from ... I had been like an uncle to him." The Vamplew family did not blame Percival and participated in the presentation of a trophy that the TTFC struck in honour of their son the following year; a younger Vamplew even ran for Percival a couple of years later, but the tragic incident could never be forgotten.

Initially, there were no females in the NTTFC and the TTFC. There were no high school track and field programs in Ontario to draw from, so many of the women who eventually joined came from backgrounds in competitive team sports such as baseball and basketball. The first woman to join the club, Shirley Eckel (Kerr), was an exception. Competing for the Toronto Malvernettes Athletic Club, an exclusively female track club, she was a member of the 4×110 yard relay team that finished first in the U.S. Nationals in 1946 and second in 1947. In 1949, she asked her coach to teach her the hurdles but was informed that at five foot, she was too short. Eckel retired for one year but returned to track and field as a member of the TTFC because Percival promised to make her into a hurdler. By 1952, Shirley Eckel was the best female hurdler in Canada and on the eve of the Olympics, she registered the second fastest time in the world.

Eckel believed strongly that Percival's coaching success was based on both his "remarkable sensitivity to body mechanics," and on the way he treated his athletes. While Percival talked about the hurdling technique he introduced to compensate for her short stature. Eckel appreciated much more his "incredible psychological approach." He understood that it would not help to tell her to "put your left elbow here." Instead she recalls, "he'd say to me, 'you must feel like a swan' and that got through to me." Eckel also remembers that "it was quite remarkable. He never talked down to a kid – he never scolded. If an error was made, it was a pat on the back and we'll do better next time."

Eckel was joined at the TTFC by another female hurdler, Gwenn Hobbins, along with sprinter Pat Jones of Vancouver, who had been on the 1948 Olympic Team and the 1950 BECG Team and was once ranked as Canada's fastest woman. The TTFC also gained a reputation for producing female athletes who excelled in the "field" part of track and field, including shot put and discus throwers Mary Lawrence, Jo Brennan and Jackie MacDonald. Mary Lawrence was gifted in many sports including basketball and baseball where she played alongside some of the women who formed the professional women's league that inspired the movie *A League of Their Own*.

Each of these women had to battle the "rigid gender stereotypes" that "discouraged women from participating in sports" at this time. These prejudices were incorporated into the AAU which deemed that while "diving, synchronized swimming, golf, tennis, gymnastics and figure skating were appropriately feminine, track and field, ice hockey, baseball, and marathon swimming were regarded as unacceptably masculine," due to their strenuous nature and the level of training they required. Jackie MacDonald recalls learning this from physical education teachers who explained that girls' activities were restricted due to fears they might do "damage to (their) reproductive organs" and that girls "weren't psychologically suited for serious competition." Fortunately, MacDonald found opportunities for competition in the community where she competed in swimming and excelled at basketball. At twenty years of age, and already employed as a schoolteacher, MacDonald discovered the shot put, the discus and Lloyd Percival.

It was not only his egalitarian ideals and scientific understanding that women could train as hard as men that inspired Percival to train so many female athletes. He also recognized that the level of women's competition in Canada was mediocre at best, and there was a tremendous opportunity to very quickly turn his protégés into champions and once again prove that his way was the right way. The young women of the TTFC did just that. Women's sports in Canada would experience serious growing pains over the next two decades. These women were in the vanguard and their coach, emerged as one of the most strident proponents of female athletics in the country.

Psychology had been a key to the success of the TTFC from the very beginning. The Red Devils nickname was intentionally provocative. Percival's choice of the colour red for the TTFC uniforms was deliberate (his mentor Knute Rockne is credited as one of the first to use colour as a psychological weapon in a major American sport). The athletes recall that their track suits were always of better quality than those worn by the other teams, and that when they warmed up in unison, it was an intimidating sight. The confidence this inspired in the TTFC athletes, and the fear it struck in the competition contributed to the remarkable success of the TTFC. As Jack McRoberts recalls, "we all believed that we could do anything we set our minds to."

Today, when athletes emerge out of nowhere and start breaking records we immediately suspect foul play. Suspicion was slower to gain a foothold in Percival's time and little was known about drugs and track and field. However, after a few years of being intimidated by the TTFC athletes and finishing well behind them in races, rumours began to spread amongst the other competitors. According to one popular story, after Percival gave caffeine tablets to his runners, "they blew away the field (and) were up for twenty-four hours afterwards." Murray Gaziuk does recall a couple of training sessions when Percival gave one half of the runners caffeine citrate and the other half a placebo. Percival charted the times but did not inform the athletes of the results. Gaziuk was never given caffeine during competition. There were also stories about Percival serving beer to the underage Red Devils and allowing the TTFC athletes to direct obscenity-laced songs at the other track and field teams. Percival was also accused of forging a signature to allow an athlete to enter a race for which that athlete was ineligible. The TTFC athletes found themselves having to defend their coach. A siege mentality evolved

– Robert Fulford recalls that it began to resemble a cult – which only served to fuel the sense of superiority Percival bred in his TTFC athletes.

All former TTFC athletes categorically deny that Percival gave them drugs or alcohol or did anything to subvert the idealistic goals of sporting competition. Instead, they attest to Percival's success in imparting a philosophy of sport that balanced the British and American creeds that had informed his developing years. Percival himself explained this philosophy in his 1952 report on the "Sports College Testing Group:"

> It is important to keep in mind that in the training
> of the Testing Group athletes, the importance of
> emotional stability, good character and the general
> qualities that go to making up an emotionally,
> physically and mentally fit and responsible citizen,
> were stressed. The fact that during the five year
> operation no member of the Testing Group has
> become ineligible due to low academic standards
> indicates that success has not been accomplished
> due to over-emphasis, but rather because of a
> philosophy that believes a well-balanced life (work,
> play, study, recreation) is an important factor in
> developing top level athletic efficiency.

Perhaps beginning in 1950 with the British Empire Games in Auckland, New Zealand, where three TTFC athletes, Gord Crosby, Rich Ferguson and Ron Miller represented Canada, but certainly by the time the 1952 Olympics in Helsinki were on the horizon, Lloyd Percival was by far and away the best track and field coach in Canada. His Toronto Track and Field Club dominated every competition and it seemed a sure thing that TTFC athletes would dominate the 1952 Olympic team. According to historical precedent, Percival should have been appointed coach of the team bound for Helsinki; however, the outburst in London in 1948 had left Percival a marked man, and he had done nothing in the intervening four years to repair the damage. The cozy relationship he had developed with some of the Toronto press and their lobbying for his appointment as 1952 Olympic coach simply made him more of an anathema to COA officials. When he was passed over for the position, Percival informed the press: "such posts go to those who meet with the approval of the Canadian Olympic Association (COA) top brass – and I'm not in this category."

In June of 1952, little more than a month prior to the Olympic Games, Percival wrote an article for *New Liberty* magazine in which he called on Canadians to support their Olympians financially and emotionally before outlining why, through no fault of their own, the athletes were doomed to failure. Percival also instructed Canadians that they should demand value for their tax dollars and require their government to better prepare for the British Empire Games in 1954 and the Melbourne Olympics in 1956. He reiterated for the public the seven point program he had presented to sports officials in 1950 and demanded that the COA adopt it, or something like it, because he wrote, "there's little point in just sponsoring a boat ride every Olympic year."

At the Olympic Track and Field Trials held in Hamilton, Ontario, on June 28 and 29, 1952, NTTC stars George Lynch, Don McEwen and Rich Ferguson all came up with sub-par performances with Lynch and McEwen failing to qualify for the team. Percival was furious. He blamed their American college coaches. "Don Canham of Michigan and Francis Cretzmeyer of Iowa worried about winning the U.S. meets with the Canadian boys. But as far as the athletes' chances of winning points for Canada were concerned Canham and Cretzmeyer just didn't care," he charged. Percival liked to bask in the glory that these coaches shone upon him when they praised the quality of the athletes he developed. Now he turned on them for using the Canadians to glorify their schools instead of Canada. He proclaimed that he would "never again recommend that a Canadian schoolboy competitor enrol at a United States College" but, of course, he would. Percival may have been the first Canadian track and field coach caught in the horns of this dilemma, but he would not be the last. The only place in North America for a track and field athlete to get decent competition after high school was on the American university circuit. Unfortunately, the tremendous pressure placed on the athletes to gain points for their college and maintain their scholarship frequently compromised the athletes' goals as Canadian internationals and sometimes shortened their careers. This was an issue with which Canadian coaches continued to wrestle for decades.

Percival's anger and disappointment with the outcome of the Olympic trials was further compounded when the Olympic Team was announced on June 30. Although the TTFC contributed more than twenty percent of the team, Percival was shocked to learn that two more of his stars had been left off of the squad. Shot putter Mary Lawrence and discus thrower Jo Brennan both set national records in their events at the Olympic trials in Hamilton but were left off the team due to lack of funds. In this case, when looking for someone to blame, Percival turned to the usual suspects – the badgers.

Money was a problem for the 1952 Olympic Team. The COA had budgeted $150,000 for the games but raised only $113,972. Not only were athletes dropped from the team, those chosen were poorly supplied. They were not given any extra pins for trading, the basketball team had none of the customary gifts to exchange for those proffered by opposing teams prior to games, and the boxers resorted to setting up a laundry service in the Olympic Village called "Canadian Olympic Cleaning and Pressing." However, when it came to deciding who would go and who would be left at home, that the two athletes dropped from the track and field team were Percival's protégés was lost on no one. A group of Toronto businessmen offered to raise the money to send Lawrence and Brennan to Helsinki, but the COA advised the men that the offer could not be accepted. When Percival learned that two fencers and two yachtsmen were added to the team after the necessary funds had been raised, he cried foul. Jim Vipond of the *Globe and Mail* agreed: "either through political pressure or rank incompetence" the selection committee betrayed the trust of the COA."

Percival had been scheduled to go to Helsinki to work for the CBC but announced that he was staying home in protest. On July 16 – just three days before the Olympics were to begin – Percival called a meeting at the 496 Church Street office of "Sports College." Rosenfeld wrote that the meeting "may go a long way to explode the present smug COA setup." Percival explained that it was time because "too many are aroused by the way the COA bigwigs have imprisoned fair play," and Rosenfeld concluded her column with "up the rebels." Unfortunately for Percival, not many rebels showed up at his office.

Canadians performed woefully in the 1952 Olympics, matching its 1948 total of only three medals, one of which was claimed by canoeists Ken Lane and Don Hawgood, who had trained with Percival. Prior to the team's departure, Percival had promised, "if they (Canadian track and field athletes) win more than four or five points, I'll eat every badge (worn by Canadian officials) over there." There were no medals and Percival did not have to eat a single badge. Before the Games were over, Jim Vipond was back criticizing Canada's poor preparation and lamenting that no one in the COA or the AAU had listened to Percival. On December 31, 1952, Percival announced his retirement from track and field coaching.

When Percival decided to forego Helsinki, it left the CBC without a colour commentator. Percival recommended Don Aitken, NTTC's fine middle distance runner, as a replacement. On the flight over, Aitken was seated up front amongst the athletes. An older Canadian official, seated further back, requested that Aitken exchange seats; Aitken declined. The official repeated his request and became confrontational when Aitken again declined. Aitken asked the man what his position was with the team. Straight faced, the man informed Aitken he would be delivering mail to the Canadian athletes in the Olympic Village. In fact, he was a university professor and a friend of a COA official who had no links to any of the athletes or the athletic teams. The 1952 Canadian Olympic Committee left qualified athletes behind due to financial shortfalls and reduced those who were chosen to begging and borrowing; they sent neither a doctor nor a trainer, but they did send a mailman.

If medical staff had accompanied the Canadian team, the Olympics may have been a different experience for hurdler Shirley Eckel who had registered the second best time in the world in the 80 metre hurdles. Soon after the long flight to London followed by seventeen hours from London to Finland, Eckel was dispatched to the track and told to start training. Without the kind of preparation and advanced training methods she was used to with Percival, Eckel pulled a hamstring in that first workout. Unlike Jack Parry in 1948, she did have a coach nearby; however, he didn't believe that she was really injured and there was no Canadian doctor to examine her. Every few days, coaches asked her to try running. Finally, the night before her race, Eckel was taken to the American team doctors. She remembers six people surrounding her on the training table and one of them stating, "if you make this girl run she will be crippled for life." Eckel was deprived of her Olympic experience, and Canada missed out on one of its best chances for a medal.

Percival's retirement didn't last long. In the spring of 1953, he was back guiding the TTFC through another dominating season and aggravating track and field officials. When a misguided taxi driver caused McRoberts, Pete Sutton and Norm Williams to be late for the Canadian Schoolboy Championships in Montreal in 1953, Percival bought some time by dismantling the hurdles set up for McRoberts' event, claiming that they were improperly weighted. As AAU officials screamed at Percival, McRoberts, Sutton and Williams were spotted jumping the fence at the end of the field. Percival declared the hurdles up to standard after all. McRoberts dressed on the track as the hurdles were being reassembled and won his event. This kind of stunt was seen as poor sportsmanship by many and certainly raises questions regarding Percival's commitment to fairness for all of the competitors, but in his mind, Percival was simply ensuring that his athletes were given the opportunity to compete as he would expect any coach to do.

McRoberts also remembers a very different side of Percival at a meet in Winnipeg later that year. The TTFC athletes arrived at the stadium the day after a major storm had passed through and found the facility strewn with debris. Percival immediately dispatched the TTFC athletes with rakes and shovels to help the organizers clean up the mess; none of the other coaches sent their athletes out. Only when the facilities were ready did Percival tell his competitors to get changed and join the other competitors. McRoberts remembers how this helped the young men and women understand that it wasn't just about their event; they "had a commitment to something bigger."

While Canadian sports officials were wondering how they could rid themselves of Percival's disruptive presence, Americans were knocking on his door. In June 1953, Columbia University offered him $6,000 per year to replace retiring track and field coach Carl Merner. Percival declined. There were other offers including those from television networks ABC, CBS and NBC to purchase "Sports College" and all of its services. Percival informed the *Globe and Mail* that he wanted to finish what he had started in Canada. He said, "there's enough favourable reaction now to give me hope that the track and field industry here will eventually endorse my mouthings as more than just bally-hoo." He would wait a long time for that validation, but soon after this interview Percival received recognition from an unlikely source.

On July 24, 1953, Her Majesty Queen Elizabeth II announced the recipients of the Coronation Medal. The list included:

> Lloyd Percival, director of Sports College, for his
> work in directing the activities of the organization
> and his contributions made in the fields of physical
> fitness and athletic research.

Percival was a surprisingly modest man when it came to displaying trophies or any symbols of past accomplishments. The Coronation Medal, however, was something that he was always proud to talk about and display. England was the birthplace of his parents and the medal meant a great deal to him. It had a place of honour in his home, a place Dorothy maintains to this day. Percival's ego always required a great deal of sustenance. He got it from his athletes and their successes, and when he received it from the Queen of England, it helped sustain him during the many years that the Canadian sports establishment shunned him

Percival's ego was also fed by frequent trips to the United States. He may not have wanted to move there, but he was pleased that the Americans would listen to him and, just as importantly, that they would pay to listen to him. Often it was his expertise as an athletic trainer that prompted the invitations. In one of her columns, Bobbi Rosenfeld suggested that since Canada never sent medical and training staff to international games, Percival's standing as probably the finest athletic trainer in Canada was reason alone to choose him as a national coach. Percival had eleven requests to deliver lectures at American coaching clinics during the summer of 1954 and, in January of that year, set off to New York State to conduct three weeks of seminars on his innovative treatment for the "charley horse." Until the early 1950s, Percival followed the prevailing wisdom and treated the charley horse with aggressive massage. In 1953, he read accounts from trainers for the Phillies baseball and Eagles football teams of Philadelphia demonstrating "how the application of ice for one to two hours after a charley horse injury" would greatly aid in a quick recovery. Percival immediately began testing this treatment on members of the St. Michael's Majors. By January of 1954, he had refined the procedure, most significantly by considerably reducing the length of time that ice was applied to the injured area. He published his findings, and was invited to New York to present a paper on the subject at the annual convention of the United States National Trainers Association. In Canada, Percival was often accused of stealing his ideas; outside of Canada, he was recognized for the depth of his research and for his willingness to look at things that others took for granted.

The 1954 British Empire and Commonwealth Games

Immediately upon his return to Toronto from the National Trainers Association Convention, Percival was again embroiled in controversy. TTFC representation on the track and field team representing Canada at the 1954 British Empire and Commonwealth Games (BECG) was expected to be even stronger than it had been on the 1952 Olympic team, and Percival's appointment as head coach should have been a *fait accompli*. Instead, there was a drawn out soap opera of bungling, subterfuge and jousting egos.

The drama began simply enough. After returning from New York on the 26th or 27th of January 1954, Percival was asked by Fred Foot, on behalf of the Central Ontario Track and Field Association (COTFA), if he would accept the position of coach for the Canadian track and field team at the upcoming British Empire and Commonwealth Games – if the position was offered. Percival said yes. On January 24, Foot sent a telegram to Fred Rowell, Chairman of the National Track and Field Committee, which read "CENTRAL ONTARIO SUGGESTS PERCIVAL AS TRACK COACH BRITISH EMPIRE TEAM." That same day Rowell wired Major John Davies, President of the British Empire and Commonwealth Games Association (BECGA): "NAME TOM LORD AS MANAGER LLOYD PERCIVAL AS TRACK COACH FRANK RICHARD CALGARY FIELD COACH NOMINATED BY QUEBEC CENTRAL ONTARIO AND ALBERTA BRANCHES RESPECTIVELY." At a January 27 meeting of the BECGA in Montreal, chaired by Davies, Davies presented these appointments with an added phrase: after the words "Lloyd Percival as Track Coach" **'not head coach'** was written in bold letters. Presumably it was Davies who added the caveat, but the origin was never explained. From this point on the whole affair became more and more convoluted.

On January 28, before any official announcement could be made, Bobbi Rosenfeld wrote in the *Globe and Mail* that sources at the Montreal meeting had advised her that Percival would "likely be named coach of Canada's lopers and leapers in the British Empire Games in Vancouver in July." When she gave Percival the news he said, "if and when it becomes official I'll be very glad. I'll strive to my utmost and do everything to make them pleased that they appointed me." As much as Percival prided himself on being an outsider, he was constantly seeking acceptance from Canadians for his controversial work. When Rosenfeld retracted her statements the following day and explained that Percival was only to be a co-coach, it was a serious blow to his ego.

Percival hid his disappointment and told Rosenfeld that he "would be pleased to help the BEGA in any way. ...But as a partial coach I don't feel I can do a proper job." He added that he had already accepted a position working for the CBC in Vancouver. They would be willing to release him if his "contribution at the British Empire Games was an important one," but not if he were "going along just as one of the boys." This indicated that pride was not the only thing driving Percival. He had no interest in going to Vancouver simply to join in the badger games, and, indeed, he could not afford to do so. He had "Sports College" to run and a wife to support. If he couldn't make a difference in Vancouver, at least he would get paid.

On his return to Vancouver, Davies was shocked to learn what had been printed in the Toronto newspapers regarding coaching decisions that were still to be officially announced. Telegrams were finally sent to the appointees and Percival wired his formal reply to Rowell on January 30:

> HONOURED TO BE SELECTED TRACK
> COACH THANKS FOR NOMINATION
> HOWEVER PREVIOUS COMMITMENTS

CBC CREATING DIFFICULT SITUATION
THOSE CONCERNED AGREE ON MY
RELIEF IN VIEW OF IMPORTANT
CONTRIBUTION I COULD MAKE ARE
NOW RELUCTANT QUESTIONS RE MY
AVAILABILITY BY FOOT SAID HEAD
COACH ACTED ACCORDINGLY NOW
VERY EMBARRASSED BY SITUATION
WHAT IS EXACT SITUATION YOUR END
REGARD LP.

No one knew quite what to do. People just didn't turn down these appointments and here was Percival, who was no favourite of any of the committee members and who, according to their private correspondence, was given the position in order to "insure good press in Toronto" making the BEG officials look bad in Eastern Canada. Telegrams flew back and forth amongst Davies, Rowell, Foot and Percival over the next five days; angry words were spoken and ultimatums delivered. When the dust had settled, all agreed that Percival should be formally named Head Coach, and he indicated that he would accept. Unfortunately, events that had been proceeding with surprising alacrity, considering the distance and the communication modes of the time, suddenly ground to a halt. When Percival finally received word from the BECGA committee that they had ratified his appointment as Head Coach, almost seven weeks had passed and all of the principals were fully aware that he would decline. Percival informed Rowell of his decision in a telegram that same day where he cited his obligations to the CBC and "Sports College" as the reason and concluded:

THIS IS A DEEP DISAPPOINTMENT TO ME
AND WISH TO EXPRESS MY REGRETS IF
I CAN BE OF ANY HELP IN AN ADVISORY
CAPACITY WILL BE DELIGHTED TO
SERVE ANY WAY TIME ALLOWS WRITING
REGARDS LP.

There is nothing in any of Percival's correspondence that betrays anything more than embarrassment and disappointment. Through it all, he hid whatever anger and disappointment he felt and presented an entirely professional attitude. Still, logic says that he should have accepted the position he so coveted. The CBC would certainly have released him if he had asked and, no matter how attractive or even necessary the money was to him, Percival never made a decision based solely on money. There were times in his life, however, when bitterness and a sense of betrayal clouded his thinking. This may have been one of them. The fact that the BECGA had gone to so much trouble, only to be rebuffed, increased their anger with Percival more than ever.

Percival expressed his true feelings by again resigning as head coach of the TTFC before the track and field season began. This time he also disbanded the club. He continued to help coach his athletes unofficially, but those who competed in Vancouver were listed as "unattached." It was a harsh blow to many athletes who depended on Percival and the suddenness of the announcement, two years after his previous angry retirement, reinforced the reputation he had gained for being selfish and egotistical and helped spawn the myth that Percival established and then disbanded numerous track clubs. According to Paul Poce, at the TTFC meeting called to announce his retirement, Percival went so far as to ask his athletes to boycott the British Empire Games on his behalf "to show the establishment that we support each other." Poce is well respected in the track and field community and claims to bear no animosity toward Percival. His story has become part of the official history of the founding of the Toronto Olympic Club (TOC); however, it was completely out of character for Percival, as egotistical, combative, pugnacious and even paranoid as he sometimes became when he was pushed, to ever ask his athletes to sacrifice all of their hard work and effort to support his ego. So many of these athletes have testified that, while they were certainly aware of his prodigious ego, Percival always put their needs ahead of his own, and they could never imagine him seriously saying such a thing. In contrast to Poce's contention, Mary Lawrence recalls Percival advising her in 1953, "You might stand a better chance of making the BECG team if you divorce yourself from me, because they don't like me." Furthermore, the published history of the TOC, which leans heavily on Poce's records and recollections of the early years, undermines his claim by stating that Poce founded the TOC on January 7, 1954, "in an effort to avoid the turmoil" caused by Percival's demands three weeks before the controversy regarding coaching selection for the BECG even began.

Percival won an award for his work with the CBC in Vancouver, which included the radio call of the Miracle Mile, in which the first two sub-four minute milers went head to head and Bannister bested Landy in one of the most famous sporting events of all time. Almost unnoticed was the remarkable third-place finish of Canada's Rich Ferguson, the TTFC runner who had become an All-American at the University of Iowa. His time of 4:04.6 was a full ten seconds faster than the previous Canadian record and would stand until Bruce Kidd broke it in 1962. It was Percival who had developed Ferguson's talent and, although Canadians were quick to credit Ferguson's American university coach, Percival would later discuss the details of the specific interval training that he had used to prepare Ferguson for the epic race.

Officially, Percival and Ferguson had nothing to do with each other at the Games. BECG officials had advised Percival not to talk to any of the thirteen TTFC athletes who were on the team, and the athletes were warned "in no uncertain terms" to stay away from him. Mary Lawrence and Jackie MacDonald remember clearly that the athletes were called together and told "a certain man has come to town – you have coaches assigned to you – don't associate with this man." The *Globe and Mail* printed this story and the BEGC made no secret of it, although they were careful not to mention Percival by name. Jack McRoberts believes that he, as well as others from TTFC, did not perform as well as they should have in Vancouver because "we knew that the guy we relied on, the guy we talked to, the guy who was our inspiration, was off limits."

For Jackie MacDonald, the association with Percival turned out to be much more problematic. MacDonald was immensely talented. She was also tall, blonde and beautiful. Percival was never shy about promoting her physical attributes and was more than pleased to use her to market track and field as a spectator sport, as well as a sport for all women. In Vancouver, the BECG was just as pleased to use her good looks to their advantage in promotions. MacDonald became a favourite of the photographers, but one photograph completely changed her life. She had already won a silver medal in the shot put when she, along with other TTFC athletes, was invited to a reception hosted by Crush Beverages, one of "Sports College's" principal sponsors and an official sponsor of the 1954 BECG. At the reception, MacDonald was photographed standing beside a Crush executive; both were holding a bottle of Orange Crush and they jointly held up a "Sports College" publication with the Crush logo on it. With MacDonald's permission, the picture appeared in the *Vancouver News Herald* the following day under a banner that read: "SPORTS COLLEGE GRADUATE" and was accompanied by text that referred to Orange Crush as a sponsor of "Sports College" and "the only soft drink chosen for the BEG stands." MacDonald did not receive payment for the advertisement and therefore did not violate any amateur rules. In addition, that same newspaper had printed an advertisement for a Persian rug company featuring a photograph of "the entire Pakistan team sitting on a rug," and "a large smiling picture of Dr. Roger Bannister," graced an advertisement for a Vancouver shoe salon.

On the morning that she was favoured to win another medal in the discus, Jackie MacDonald was summoned to a meeting with Margaret Lord, Chaperone of the Women's track and field team, and Hy Herschorn, Vice-President of the BECGA. "I didn't have a clue what it was about," she recalls. "One team official – a lawyer (Herschorn) – called a witness in and locked the door. ... It was nasty. … They really gave me the third degree – about Lloyd – I don't think they even mentioned Orange Crush." MacDonald was barred from her event and had to await another hearing to determine if she had violated her amateur oath. Even though the final ruling cleared her of any wrongdoing, the spokesperson for the BECG stated that the "committee recognizes that the action taken on Miss MacDonald was proper to protect the athletes and other nations in the Games, until her position was clarified."

MacDonald believed then, and is even more convinced today, that she was punished because of her association with Percival. One official rather indiscreetly "admitted this to a newsman at a dance following the Games." So offended was the BEGC by Percival's mere presence in Vancouver that they felt compelled to make special reference to him in their official report published following the Games, complaining, in spite of testimony to the opposite from the former TTFC athletes, about "interference in training routine by outside coaches…one man proved himself to be a particularly objectionable type and constantly broke his word to us."

Retirement and Reflection

This time Percival did not rescind his retirement. Track and field officials all across Canada were happy that he was gone, but they could not erase the phenomenal record of his NTTFC-TTFC track clubs. They had won virtually every team title in every track meet they entered and were so dominant that the 289 points they tallied in the 1953 Ontario Track and Field Championships were more than 200 points better than the next best club. By 1954, TTFC athletes had won 2,500 medals, including 1,000 gold, established more than 500 city, provincial and national records and won more than 1,600 individual championships in every event except the hammer throw. The Viscount Alexander Award, honouring the best junior track and field athlete in Canada, went to a TTFC member in five out of the seven years it was presented. The group that Percival took to Madison Square Garden in 1952 gained more points than any American school team in the competition, and thirty-nine TTFC athletes earned scholarships to American universities.

Furthermore, Percival had changed the culture of track and field in Ontario. He challenged his athletes and made them believe that they could defeat anyone, spearheaded most of the innovation and change that occurred in Ontario track and field, and it was the success of his athletes that forced other coaches to modernize their coaching methods. He established Ontario as a breeding ground for great athletic talent. No longer was it good enough to simply win local races. Ontario coaches and athletes began to believe that they could compete with athletes from south of the border, and their success paved the way for many more Canadians to gain scholarships to American universities.

Many of the TTFC scholarship recipients overshadowed the Americans at their schools. Don McEwan and George Lynch at the University of Michigan and Rich Ferguson at the University of Iowa held NCAA records; Ferguson and McEwan won NCAA championships. Some did well in spite of being surprised at how little their university coaches knew. Murray Cockburn discovered that the distance runners at USC didn't receive much coaching: "they just brought in a bunch of guys who fought it out for positions on the team." Cockburn developed his own program through correspondence with Percival and shared the program with other USC runners. His was not a unique situation.

More importantly, all of the young men Percival helped earn scholarships – scholarship opportunities for women were extremely limited and did not extend to Canadians – gained scholastic standing and life experience that would otherwise have been quite different for some and completely out of reach for others. Examples are Don Aitken, whose injuries led him to exchange his athletic scholarship for an academic scholarship and a master's degree, and Charles (Chuck) Tobias, who stayed in the United States after graduating from USC. Today, he owns Pusser's Rum and his own island paradise and reflects, "I owe a huge amount of my success to him (Percival) – more than to anyone else in my life."

There were also TTFC athletes who chose Canadian universities including Murray Gaziuk who won national championships while competing for the University of Toronto. After graduation, he became a teacher and a principal, a track and field coach and an administrator, was named to the National Advisory Council for Fitness and Amateur Sport and helped start ParticipACTION. Gaziuk was unequivocal in his praise: "It all comes back to Lloyd – the love of sport and the love of competition."

Ron Miller is one of those who did not go to university. Percival helped make him Canada's best pole vaulter, a member of the 1952 Olympic team and a silver medalist at the 1954 British Empire Games. Miller attended art school after retiring from sports and became a successful photographer. He credits Percival with giving him "an inspiration and a drive to achieve." Without Percival's training, Gord Crosby would not have run the high hurdles at the 1952 Olympics. Crosby had grown up a ward of the Children's Aid Society and admitted to having "some problems getting along with people." Percival gave him some books to read and talked to him a great deal about life. Crosby went into sales and soon owned his own car dealership. Crosby is thankful that Percival "was not only a good coach, he helped us in life."

Percival's work with young men like Crosby was noted by two lawyers who asked if he could work with some of the boys at the Whitby Training School, a residential facility east of Toronto for minors in trouble with the law. Roy Beaumont was one of the boys Percival helped. Beaumont had a difficult childhood, had learned to talk later than most, did not attend school and could neither read nor write. It took a while, but Lloyd and Dorothy convinced Beaumont to attend adult literacy classes. The classes proved so successful that when he learned that Jackie MacDonald was a school teacher, Beaumont asked her to be his private tutor. The Children's Aid Society paid for the sessions. With MacDonald's assistance, Roy

Beaumont completed his courses and graduated from the Ryerson Polytechnic apprenticeship program. He then embarked on a successful career as a plumber, eventually owning his own plumbing company.

Beaumont and the other TTFC athletes frequently visited the Percival home on Glen Road. Joan Sutton wrote about Percival many times after she became a columnist with the *Toronto Telegram*, and later the *Toronto Sun*, but she first met Lloyd and Dorothy when she was dating her future husband, TTFC member, Pete Sutton. In fact, she only became sure that Pete was serious about their relationship after he took her to Glen Road to meet the Coach one Sunday. The weekly Sunday night get-togethers are the times best remembered by the former Red Devils. Dorothy always cooked for the boys, looked after their injuries and listened to their troubles. Lloyd, too, had a sympathetic ear, but he was usually busy regaling them with stories, discussing team strategy and building their confidence for the upcoming meet. Everyone felt at home in the Percival house. Sutton remembered that "They offered warmth, understanding and, for many, a foothold on life." Of Roy Beaumont, Sutton wrote, "Lloyd took him in, Do (Dorothy) mothered him and he became a useful member of society." She added, "The kid whose father was an alcoholic, the kid whose mother was a prostitute, all found a sense of worth in the world of the Percivals."

Other Sports

Lacrosse

JIM BISHOP WAS A COACHING PRODIGY. Like Percival, Bishop was just seventeen years old when he took over the reins of a peewee team named the Toronto's Lakeshore Golden Gaels lacrosse team. Unlike Percival, Bishop found a mentor close by. The two men began a close personal and professional relationship in 1946 and Bishop joined the "Sports College" staff in 1952. Bishop applied the same dedication to training lacrosse players that Percival applied to all of his athletes. A Jim Bishop team was always the fittest lacrosse team on the floor. He was known to be merciless, ran hard practices the afternoon of a night game and again at midnight if the team played badly. People compared Bishop to a Marine drill sergeant, but there was more to Jim Bishop's coaching, and for that, he owed a huge debt to Lloyd Percival.

In a 1969 *Toronto Star* article about Bishop and the Oshawa Green Gaels lacrosse team he had coached to seven consecutive national junior lacrosse championships, journalist Frank Orr referred to Bishop as "probably the finest coach working in any team sport in Canada." Bishop talked to Orr about the influence of Percival and stated:

> The most important thing that Percival taught me
> was the desire to find new ways of doing things. He
> taught me how I was to break down the barriers of
> learning new methods and that there was no value
> in a dogmatic attachment to the old ways.

115

The Pulford brothers played for the Green Gaels in the 1950s when the team was based in Toronto and in Newmarket. Bob Pulford, a member of the last Toronto Maple Leaf team to win the Stanley Cup, was also a coach and an executive in the NHL, while Clarke became one of the most respected coaches and administrators in the history of Toronto high school sports. Both remember Bishop's tough training sessions as well as those occasions when Percival was there to run the team through physical and psychological tests.

Charles Bull was a teammate of the Pulfords. When he was thirteen years old, he became acquainted with Percival through the *Sports College News*. While playing for the Green Gaels, Bull attended medical school and a natural bond was formed with Percival. The relationship was renewed in the 1960s after Bull graduated and became one of Canada's first sports medicine specialists. Dr. Bull recalls one occasion when Percival tested the players to see how long each could hold their breath. Ostensibly, it was a physiological test, but Percival liked to use it to determine an athlete's psychological strength. On this particular day, Dr. Bull remembers holding his breath for one and one-half minutes, due to his training as a competitive swimmer, while Clarke Pulford could manage only forty-five seconds. Percival lectured the boys on how, with determination, they could double their time before asking them to try again. Bull could not appreciably improve his time, but, on his second attempt, Pulford held his breath for one minute before collapsing on the floor. Bull remembers Percival enthusiastically declaring Pulford the winner "because he was the most determined" and stating that "all of us should have passed out." Percival knew that this would not harm the boys, and it was one of the many ways he taught his athletes that sport was very much mind over matter. There was another aspect of his work with the Green Gaels that was more controversial. Dr. Bull remembers, "One time he (Percival) had us take caffeine pills (half took a pill with caffeine and half took one without)." Dr. Bull explains that he was "hyper" anyway, and the pills threw off his timing. Percival told him that he didn't need any pills, "that they were better for the big defencemen." Another Green Gaels also recalls that caffeine pills were taken by players on the team but did not relate it directly to Bishop or Percival and wished not to elaborate. Caffeine was not a banned substance. The incident described by Dr. Bull was a controlled test – as was the one reported by Murray Gaziuk of the Red Devils – and is consistent with Percival's scientific approach to sport. While we have no other testimony to Percival's providing caffeine to athletes, the fact that he was known to have tested the effects of caffeine on his athletes helped spawn rumours of widespread drug use amongst Percival's track and field competitors.

Canoeing

One of the qualities that sets Lloyd Percival apart from any other coach in Canadian history and grants him an honoured position in any worldwide hierarchy of athletic coaches was his ability to take the scientific, psychological and practical knowledge he gathered from his many contacts throughout the sports world, as well as through "Sports College" and the "Sports College testing group", and transfer that knowledge to a wide range of sports and physical activities. His track and field athletes certainly benefited from the encyclopaedic knowledge he continued to accrue, and we have seen how he applied his knowledge of modern scientific training in track and field to his work with hockey and lacrosse players. However, when two canoeists came to him in late 1951, this process of grafting knowledge gained in one sport onto the training programs he devised for athletes in completely different sports was advanced to yet another level.

In August 1951, Ken Lane and Don Hawgood of Toronto were chosen to represent Canada in the 10,000 metre two-man canoe event – known as the Canadian Pairs or C2 – at the 1952 Olympics in Helsinki. That the canoeing contingent to be sent to Helsinki was selected in 1951 was in itself progressive. Percival complained throughout the 1950s about the:

Totally ridiculous system whereby we are caught
up in a last-minute flurry just before Games
time every four years, trying to scrape together a
team made up of athletes who, even giving their
best, could not hope to carry away an Olympic
crown, simply because they haven't been given the
opportunity and background to come through such
a demanding test.

Percival credited only the Swimming and Canoeing Federations as being strong enough to act independently of the COA. In the case of canoeing, this meant selecting a team in late summer when they had peaked for their National Championships instead of in the spring when they would be better off building slowly for the Olympic Games.

Lane and Hawgood approached Percival because of his reputation as a good track and field coach. The tandem partners were thirty-one and thirty-five years old respectively, advanced in age for competitive canoeing. They knew it would be their last Olympics and wanted to ensure that they were in the best possible condition. Percival designed a program of stretching and light weights for the winter and arranged for Lane and Hawgood to workout at Toronto's Mayfair Club on their lunch hours. He also recommended numerous changes in their diet. Sugar was largely eliminated as were coffee and black tea. Lane and Hawgood were advised to substitute Ovaltine and green tea – almost fifty years before green tea was championed in the west. Percival was also in that small cadre who were adamant about the benefits of vitamins. In this case, it was vitamin C. In the absence of the concentrated tablets available today, Lane and Hawgood were asked to eat as many as three oranges with every meal and had to order them by the case from a wholesaler.

The Royal Canadian Yacht Club (RCYC) offered the paddlers bound for Helsinki a training base on Toronto Island. Percival began spending weekends there with Art Johnson and Tom Hodgson, who were to compete in the C2 1,000 metres, Bert Oldershaw who was competing in the single kayak (K1) and Doug Bennet and Harry Poulton who were preparing for the tandem kayak (K2), but he devoted extra time to Lane and Hawgood

Clear to Percival from the beginning was the requirement for tremendous endurance in a race that lasted almost one hour; however, when Lane and Hawgood explained to Percival how the 10,000 metre race took place on the 1,000 metre course and required nine turns around buoys marking the end of the course and that twenty-six crews competed for space on an eleven lane course, Percival gained an appreciation of how race strategy would influence training. He developed a program that maximized the canoeists' ability to get off to a fast start but also enable them to change pace at will and put in surges. That way, if Lane and Hawgood failed to emerge from the mass start at the head of the pack, they would still be able to pick off crews and gain the first corner before any other tandem. Percival also convinced the tandem that if they sprinted out of each turn they would gain a physical and psychological advantage over crews still struggling through the slow corner.

Not one canoeist in the world was known to have attempted this strategy, but Percival was aware of a similar approach taken by Emil Zatopek in track and field. The tremendous volume of interval training done by Zatopek not only gave him the strength and stamina to dominate his events, it also allowed him to toy with his opponents and wear them down physically and mentally by routinely changing pace. Percival had already introduced interval training to his distance runners and had suggested it to the Detroit Red Wings. In the on-the-water program drawn up for Lane and Hawgood, he applied the same scientific principles.

Lane and Hawgood would put in two hour sessions of 200 metre hard intervals with 100 metre easy recoveries between intervals. Percival was frequently on-site, timing the sessions and gauging the progress of the pair. At the end of one session when the partners were particularly exhausted, Percival exhorted them to go all out for another 500 metres. When, to their amazement, they managed to power their boat right through the finish line, Lane recalls Percival explaining to them that when their mind was telling them that they couldn't do it, it was really just a warning that they were approaching their limit. Lane, who later became Ontario Seniors Squash champion, said he learned from Percival that for an athlete to become a champion, he must be able to overcome "the mind's attempt to protect the body."

In Helsinki, the canoe and kayak races were held in the capricious waters of Helsinki Harbour where waves coming through the gaps in the breakwall sometimes reached six feet. This played havoc with many crews including Johnson and Hodgson who were disqualified from a heat after a wave pushed them out of their lane. This was unfortunate since Percival had clocked the pair on Toronto Island at times that would have placed them amongst the medal winners. Bert Oldershaw (grandfather of Mark Oldershaw, the 2012 Olympic bronze medalist in the 1,000 Metre C1) reached the finals and finished ninth, the best placing by a Canadian kayak paddler prior to 1992.

Lane and Hawgood followed Percival's race plan to the letter. After a series of surges, they rounded the 1,000 metre buoy in first place, closely followed by a strong French crew that was not intimidated by the surges Lane and Hawgood initiated coming out of every corner. In fact, the French employed their own clever strategy, saving valuable energy by riding the wake of the Canadian boat. The two crews were locked this way until they came out of the final turn, and the French crew swung wide. Since there were only two widely separated buoys to mark the finish line in the open bay, it was very difficult to pick the best line to the finish. The French crew found the shortest route and it came down to a photo finish. After five minutes of studying the pictures, France was awarded the Gold Medal, Canada the Silver; the third place Russians were more than eight minutes behind. The silver medal won by Lane and Hawgood was one of only three medals won by Canadians in Helsinki. None of the canoeists were charged a cent for Percival's time and effort;

Lane and Hawgood were not even asked to pay dues to the Mayfair Club even though they spent almost every lunch hour working out there from August 1951 until they left for Helsinki in August 1952.

Research Studies, Publications and Government Policy

NO MATTER HOW INVOLVED PERCIVAL BECAME in helping paddlers prepare for the Olympics, developing training programs for lacrosse teams or studying Russian hockey, he always made sure that he had a good script prepared for "Sports College of the Air" each Saturday along with exploring interesting ideas for "Sports College" publications. Save for a temporary switch to a 6:30 p.m. Saturday time slot and the introduction of more material directed at females and adults, the very successful format of "Sports College of the Air" remained constant and the catalogue of publications continued to grow.

The 1953 "Sports College" catalogue contained thirty-five titles; by 1957, there were sixty-three. In addition, "Sports College" offered a list of fifty books by other authors "analyzed, approved and recommended as tops in their field." Also available through mail order were "Sports College" crests, pennants, tie clips, T-shirts and sets of York Weights. The vast majority of the new "Sports College" publications were straightforward and fiscally, as well as physically, economical discussions of nutrition, health, fitness and all manner of sports. There were a few publications that utilized more innovative techniques for interesting young people and coping with problems of space and portability. For example, the four booklets in the Bulletin "C" Series on hockey, printed on heavy gauge, brightly coloured construction paper with photographs and drawings, were particularly attractive and durable. Since one featured Gordie Howe and his tips on goal scoring and another presented Red Kelly's advice on playing defence, these were designed for young people to cherish and save.

A particularly innovative approach to presenting information is found in the "How To" series produced after 1957 which included *How to be a Track and Field Champion*. What appears to be a simple four page pamphlet (counting front and back covers) created using a birthday card format accomplished by folding an 11 inch by 8 ½ inch piece of heavy gauge paper once was actually an 11 inch by 17 inch page folded twice. After reading the four pages immediately visible in the booklet, the reader could find an equal amount of information on the inner 11 inch by 17 inch page when opened up. This is an ingenious presentation of 5,000 words of detailed instructions on sprints, middle and long distance running, hop step and jump, broad jump, pole vault, shot put, discus, high jump, javelin, hurdles and general track and field hints. With the support of excellent graphics, Percival provided any track and field coach with the basic tools to teach all disciplines of the sport.

Percival's modern attitude towards women in sport had been outlined in the very first issue of the *Sports College Research Guide (SCRG)* in 1951, where he devoted a full page to debunking the myth that women's bodies were not designed for sports. He quoted international research, supported by "Sports College" studies begun at the Olympics in London in 1948, in contending that "continued participation in sport should improve a girl's figure, not destroy it." Percival argued that more Canadian women and girls active in sport would mean:

- A fitter nation: (More men would also take part.)

- More happy husbands and boyfriends: (The "sports widow" would be a person of the past.)

- More youths interested in sports: (The influence of the mother.)

- A more personable Canadian woman: (Because of a better rounded personality and figure – more vitality and basic fitness.)

Still, Percival's writings at the time also reflect a largely traditional view that fitness for women was especially important for improving and maintaining physical appearances. Consequently, articles were devoted to enhancing the bust line, and an eight page, 8 ½ inch by 11 inch booklet with a pretty blue cover featuring an attractive woman in a bathing suit was devoted to B*uilding Beautiful Legs*.

A similarly designed but more sombre booklet published in the late 1950s was entitled *Fitness for Smokers*. Percival was clear and emphatic in his anti-smoking message to the Detroit Red Wings and all other athletes but was a life-long smoker himself. Like many smokers, Percival quit and started again many times and would cut back only to increase his consumption again. It was one of the things that people who met him found incongruous. He often informed people that he smoked in order to test his theories on himself. In reality he was addicted and by publishing a booklet titled *Fitness for Smokers* with the caveat: "This is not approval of smoking but a realistic guide designed to offset, as much as possible, its possible harmful effects on health and fitness levels." Percival was dealing with the reality that many people smoked. He was attempting to use exercise and proper nutrition to assist smokers in becoming as healthy as possible. The *Toronto Telegram* supported his efforts by publishing two articles based on *Fitness for Smokers* in June 1959.

This may seem anachronistic in this day and age except that an article titled "Hack and Field" appeared in the *National Post* on February 7, 2007. It tells the story of the president of a very successful track club, which specializes in training marathon runners, discovering some of his best athletes secretly indulging their smoking habits on the night of the club's annual banquet. In her exploration of the psychological and physiological implications of smoking for the physically fit, the author quotes contemporary researchers who suggest that "increased physical activity (for smokers) is associated with reduction in the risk of cardiovascular diseases and several types of cancers and an increase in active life expectancy." This is exactly what Percival told his readers in 1958.

Percival believed that it was better to work with the realities of society rather than ignore them; that even a small step forward was better than no step at all. When he concluded that modern man was becoming "deskbound" and was committing "armchair suicide," Percival devised a series of light exercises that could be performed while seated at a desk. Just as he accepted that some people would continue to smoke, Percival acknowledged that there were those who were going to sit at their desk all day. Yes, it would be better if they went for a run at lunch time, but if they weren't about to, they could at least do these simple exercises. Academics scoffed at such programs, but Percival didn't care. He was interested in improving the lives of anyone and everyone. As he stated so often, fitness could but would not necessarily "add years to your life." However, fitness would most definitely "add life to your years." Furthermore, Percival was possessed by an apostolic faith that once people were exposed to the benefits of fitness and a healthy diet, they would continue to exercise in some form or other and would adopt a more healthy diet.

During the 1950s, Percival and "Sports College" published a number of important research studies which examined the fitness of Canadians, how much they understood about fitness and if improving their fitness could improve their lives. Out of these studies came four "Sports College" publications, each containing fifty to one hundred pages and selling for $1.00 a piece: *RELAXATION is easy* (1954); *Fitness is Easy: A Basic Fitness Program for Canadians* (1957); *How to Stay Slim and Healthy* (1957); and *Fitness for Your Children* (1958). These four books, along with the 1949 submission to the Massey Commission, the 1950 *Report to the Detroit Red Wings* and the 1951 *Hockey Handbook* constitute the major canons in Percival's gospel on health, fitness and sport.

RELAXATION is easy is "the first sport psychology book ever written" according to Dr. Thomas Tutko, the father of sport psychology. There were clinical psychologists, such as Coleman Griffith, dabbling in sports prior to Dr. Tutko's ground-breaking work at San Jose State University in the 1960s, but they were interested in analyzing theoretical concepts. Dr. Tutko pioneered the study of how psychology directly impacts upon athletic performance and how an understanding of psychology can be used to improve performance. The books he published including *Problem Athletes and How to Handle them* (1966) written with Dr. Bruce Ogilvie, and *Winning is Everything and Other American Myths* (1976) are classics in the field, but it is Percival's 1954 publication, *RELAXATION is easy* that Dr. Tutko recognized as the original.

RELAXATION is easy is designed to help the athlete, the businessman, the coach, the housewife, parents or "anyone who must operate under any kind of pressure." The book begins:

> Try this ...
>
> Put your hand out in front of you. Hold your breath and clench your fist. Now – exhale slowly and let your hand fall open limply.
>
> That, fundamentally, is all you have to do to learn how to relax ...
>
> Relaxation is a simple, neuromuscular skill.

Percival identified two kinds of tension:

1. Affective (Muscular) tension is caused by anxiety and is to a large degree unconsciously created.

2. Co-ordination tension is caused (1) by incorrect use of the muscles when the person goes into action or (2) by his determination to play harder or better.

The causes of the two types are different, but the effect is "much the same," a "tightening of the muscles which is not necessary."

The first type of tension affects everyone to some degree or another: a salesman making a pitch, anyone giving a speech, a singer with stage fright, or an athlete before the big game. All experience anxiety that can ebb and flow as situations change. Co-ordination tension is more particular to sports. Percival explained that for each group of muscles in the body there is another group that balances it. "If a movement is to be made efficiently, only the muscles concerned must go into action, the others must remain relaxed." This is why a golfer trying too hard to hit it over the pond, a baseball player trying to hit a home run or a sprinter tensing up to drive out of the blocks is doomed to failure because "their movements are restricted because the counter muscles are in action too."

Percival believed that in order for someone to be able to recognize tension, he or she had to develop a clear understanding of what tension felt like. He instructed readers on how to create tension, how to feel what it was like to be engaged by it, how to consciously release it and how to appreciate the change. Once the reader had grasped "recognition control," he or she could use the drills that targeted specific parts of the body. In this way, it was similar to a yoga practice. Just as in yoga, breathing exercises were considered essential and a sort of daily meditation practice was offered as the final element. Percival never admitted to anything more than a rudimentary knowledge of yoga; however, many of the drills and relaxation techniques, including exercises for the eyes, bare a remarkable similarity in design and in purpose to yoga asanas. The book systematically leads one through a physical and psychological journey. Furthermore, the name Percival gave to a chest building exercise he had first introduced in the August 30, 1952, "Sports College" program, "Ghandi Chest Puffs" (a variation of the Baddha Konasana, or Cobbler's Pose), suggests that Percival's debt to this ancient Eastern practice was greater than he admitted.

Percival offered many examples of athletes who, while fully capable of peak performance in practice, repeatedly failed in competition. He countered this with examples of great athletes such as Gordie Howe and Roger Bannister who "make things look easy." The 3:59.4 mile that Roger Bannister ran just prior to the publication of *RELAXATION is easy* was presented as the greatest example of sustained relaxation in the face of unbelievable pressure. Many gifted middle distance runners had flirted with the sub-four minute mile, but none had seriously threatened to break it. The interval training credited with giving runners the necessary physical capability had been understood by the best track and field coaches since 1950, and the possibility of a sub-four minute mile and who would be the first to run it was the subject of much conjecture. It is interesting to note that in May 1951, the *Globe and Mail* quoted Percival as saying that Bannister would be the first because Percival had watched the British miler run a 56.7 second final quarter-mile at the Penn Relays "without signs of strain." Percival spoke with Bannister at the 1954 British Empire Games in Vancouver, three months after he had run the first sub-four minute mile. Bannister explained to Percival that his ability to relax was "one of the main secrets of peak performance" and described what we now refer to as visualization techniques.

RELAXATION is easy is masterfully written. Between its covers can be found more practical information on the psychology of sport than was included in any psychology text until Dr. Tutko and his protégés entered the field a dozen years later. According to Dr. Tutko, Percival employed a "personal, accepting manner" to present the athlete, the coach and the parent with a "unified support system that was unique." Furthermore, Dr. Tutko said that the book offered the non-athlete a "fresh means of coping with everyday life." This was essential not only to this book, but to almost everything Percival wrote. He saw increased tension as one of the most dangerous products of modern society. In a warning that has been substantiated by modern medical research, he wrote in *RELAXATION is easy* that tension:

> Creates discomfort, irritation and interferes with the proper functioning of the body and will, if long continued, cause illness and disease. It is something that everyone should learn to avoid or control. It is one of the greatest enemies of mankind.

If there is one of these four "Sports College" publications that sits at the centre of Percival's philosophical universe, it is *Fitness is Easy*. Percival grew up in a social milieu where physical fitness itself was not an objective. People engaged in sporting activities, not to improve their level of fitness, but for the social involvement and to satisfy a basic human need for competition. For the most part, they were correct in assuming that their ordinary daily activities were sufficient to keep them fit enough to live a healthy life. Sporting fitness was a luxury for those who wanted it. By the eve of WWII, society had changed. The discovery that fully one third of Canadian males were unfit for military service pushed the post-war government into its limited role of promoting health and fitness, but the government made it clear that its purpose was to ensure military preparedness for the future. In the public consciousness, the association between fitness and health was still extremely tenuous.

By 1950, Canada had entered an unprecedented era of post-war prosperity based on urbanization and rapid technological change. Percival was one of many who worried that the transition from an agrarian and blue collar economy, where manual labour was a way of life, to a more urban and white collar working class, where machines relieved society of much of life's natural physical challenge, was leading to dangerously low fitness levels. He wrote: "What our forefathers got naturally because of their need for physical activity to live in their environment we must now develop purposefully." There were a number of well-publicized research studies published in Europe and the United States that dealt with this problem. Since Percival wanted to gain a measure of physical fitness amongst Canadians, he initiated his own "Sports College" studies.

In 1952, Percival released the initial results of a "National Fitness Study" of 10,000 Canadians who voluntarily answered a "Sports College" questionnaire along with the results of physical testing performed by "Sports College" staff on a much smaller sample of volunteers. In April 1953, *Maclean's* magazine printed a feature story written by Percival on the results of his study. It led with a banner:

> LLOYD PERCIVAL, Director of Sports College
> says OUR FLABBY MUSCLES ARE
> A NATIONAL DISGRACE

The article outlined the findings of the "Sports College" survey and compared them to results of similar tests conducted in Europe and Australia. It also included a fifteen step home fitness test with explanatory photographs. As the banner suggests, Percival pulled no punches. He argued that Canada's dismal performance at the 1948 Olympics – 24th place amongst competing nations – stemmed from the inferior fitness level of the average Canadian citizen. But in his analysis of the causes and in his suggested solutions, Percival focused his attention not on Olympic athletes but on the improvement of the everyday lives of Canadians. The dire situation described by Percival, such as the warnings regarding obesity and the declining fitness of the nation's youth, sound so familiar that the article would be at home in a *Maclean's* today.

Percival followed up the "National Fitness Test" with a "Sports College" study of 51,555 Canadians of all ages and from all walks of life who had responded to a questionnaire and either submitted to physical tests by "Sports College" staff or administered themselves the simple tests provided. He published the results in the July 1955 edition of *Sports College News*. As was generally the case with Percival's studies, the results were criticized for their lack of scientific rigour. Percival was undeterred and quoted well-known medical figures as well as similar international studies to support his claim that only 13.2% of Canadian males and 27.2% of Canadian females achieved a basic level of fitness. Rural Canadians registered much higher passing grades (72.8%) than did urban residents (12.2% town and village and 7.1% city); income and age were not found to be a determining factor. Percival also pronounced Canadians "physically illiterate" because the majority did not have a good grasp of what physical fitness was and how it impacted upon their lives.

Convinced that the declining level of physical fitness in Canada "adds up to lower life expectancy, decreased enjoyment of life, less safety, lower efficiency at work, a dulling of the senses, increased strain and tension and less reserve in case of emergencies," Percival wrote *Fitness is Easy*. While he always stressed enjoying life, as opposed to just living it, Percival wasn't averse to using people's fear of their mortality to convince them to get fit. In *Fitness is Easy*, he invoked the testimony of a dozen of the world's leading health authorities to prove that a lack of fitness w hat this was even more significant to those over forty years of age because, as Dr. Paul D. White, President Eisenhower's personal heart specialist, had said, "day by day it is becoming more and more apparent that we don't wear out – we rust out!"

After presenting the results of the "Sports College" research studies to convince readers just how unfit Canadians really were, Percival proceeded with the 'easy' part of his *Fitness is Easy* book – exercises that would remedy the problems. They were the same simple, straightforward routines that became standards of his fitness formula. In recognition of the problems of repetition and boredom, he offered alternate and supplementary exercises and short sections on nutrition, weight control, sleep, smoking, posture, mental approach, tension control and balanced living. To those who might be intimidated by exercise programs, Percival explained that even a small amount of exercise or physical work was better than none at all. Throughout the remaining years of his life, Percival would never waiver from anything laid out in this book and continued to promote it as a basic guide to healthy living for all Canadians.

Fitness is Easy marked the first time that artwork became an important component of Percival's publications. It included caricatures created by Tom Hodgson, one of Canada's most famous artists of the second half of the twentieth century – he had previously contributed to the cover of *RELAXATION is easy*. Hodgson was a member of the Olympic canoeing team that trained with Percival on Toronto Island prior to the 1952 Olympics. In 1956, Hodgson was training on his own but followed the methods he had learned from Percival and, with partner Bill Stephenson, finished ninth in the 1,000 metre C2 at the Melbourne Olympics. During these years, Hodgson provided Percival with free artwork for his publications and rendered wonderful portraits of some of the Red Devils track stars.

Hodgson's graphics notwithstanding, the most significant artistic contribution to *Fitness is Easy* comes from the accurate, anatomical drawings by Doug MacLennan, a former student at the Ontario College of Art. MacLennan was born and raised in Toronto, had a background in sports and knew of Lloyd Percival. It was at Bowling Green State University in Ohio (BGSU) where MacLennan was majoring in health and physical education and contemplating graduate studies in physiotherapy, however, that he first entertained the idea of working with Percival. One of his lecturers at BGSU distributed copies of *Sports College News* to the class, and MacLennan decided to contact Percival about possible summer employment. While home for the Christmas holidays in 1955, MacLennan visited Percival, who invited him to come back in the summer. MacLennan never enrolled in graduate school. Instead, he joined the "Sports College" staff in the summer of 1956 and gradually assumed Joe Taylor's position as Percival's "right-hand man," a position he would hold for almost twenty years. Taylor's outside editing duties eventually took him to Africa for a decade before he came back to become Percival's senior editor.

From the time that MacLennan arrived at "Sports College," the publications featured simple but pleasingly human forms that illustrated the different movements and postures required to perform various exercises described in the printed materials. Like Joe Taylor, MacLennan also wrote for "Sports College." His extensive knowledge of physiology gained through a personal training regimen that earned him the title of 'Mr. Muscles' in one of the "Sports College" promotions helped MacLennan write the myriad and diverse training programs demanded by Percival over the years. He also proved to be an excellent public speaker. Percival was an engaging orator who was in constant demand and had a habit of accepting engagements without consulting his schedule. On Doug MacLennan's first day on the job, he was sent to speak to the East York Y.M.C.A. – a "trial by fire" similar to that which Percival subjected his track and field athletes. Throughout their twenty years together, MacLennan was frequently asked to take over Percival's public speaking engagements, often on very short notice and sometimes with no notice at all. MacLennan was an excellent spokesman for "Sports College" and later The Fitness Institute, but he was not Lloyd Percival and he sympathised with the disappointment his arrival sometimes engendered.

Lloyd Percival expected a great deal from people, especially those who worked closely with him. Alan Percival, followed by Joe Taylor and Doug MacLennan, were each expected to work at the same frenetic pace as their mercurial boss and rarely saw their names appear on the final documents. That references to MacLennan, Taylor, Alan Percival and Lloyd's wife, Dorothy, who was a huge help to her husband especially in the early years, do not feature more prominently in these pages is not due to the author's failure to appreciate their contributions to the success of "Sports College" and Percival's many other projects. It is simply that Percival was the source, the inspiration and the constant in all of these activities. It is often impossible to determine how much each individual contributed to the various projects completed in Percival's name, and it is less confusing to attribute such to the man who was the inspiration and the centre of everything.

One thing is certain: Dorothy had helped her husband edit *The Hockey Handbook* and had typed the entire manuscript. The regular royalty cheques earned from the book enabled the Percival's to purchase a home at 9 Tremont Road in Don Mills in 1957. Don Mills was a new planned community in what was then the north part of Toronto, and Lloyd was something of a celebrity in his new neighbourhood. He somehow found time to serve as Chairman of the Don Mills Community Association, and one of his first projects was to initiate a fitness program which he claimed would make the citizens of Don Mills "the healthiest in all Canada." Percival never completed this program; however, as a first step, he initiated the largest (in terms of direct, personal study) and by far the most influential of all of his research studies. He named it *The Don Mills Mass Fitness Test.*

For this study, three hundred children, aged six to twelve, were put through a battery of tests that were divided into two units and administered by trained nurses and physiotherapists. The first unit consisted of "six minimum tests" designed by Dr. Hans Kraus and Dr. Sonja Weber of the Institute of Physical Medicine and Rehabilitation at New York University. The Don Mills children registered a 59% failure rate on this first unit of tests, comparable to results found when the same tests had been administered in American cities. When compared to the 9% failure rate of European children, however, the results were disturbing. The second unit was comprised of "four maximum tests" designed by "Sports College" and intended to determine if the subjects possessed "sufficient strength, flexibility, and co-ordination to lead really efficient physical lives." Percival stressed that these were not tests that only athletes would be able to pass. They were intended to assess one's ability to engage in "active living." It was this emphasis on functionality and the application to daily living that most interested Percival. It was also what separated him from the academics and social scientists and left his surveys along with the results he published the object of derision and scorn.

Only 15% of the participants reached the basic standard Percival and his "Sports College" staff set for the second unit of the *Don Mills Mass Test*. While he acknowledged that these results could not be compared to any scientific studies conducted in the United States or in Europe, Percival considered them important because they gave a measure of what he believed was the children's potential to enjoy life, not just live it. He spoke to the parents through these results when he reworked one of his favourite adages that through fitness, "the sky looks bluer, the steak tastes better, the work load feels lighter and even the mortgage payments seem easier."

Percival published the complete results of the *Don Mills Mass Test* in February 1958 along with the promise of a free Family Fitness Package designed to help all Canadians improve their level of fitness without having to leave their own homes. Percival was a master at getting attention from the media, but this time he outdid himself. It was a catch phrase he coined that caught the attention of reporters and publishers across Canada, the United States and even Europe. Percival referred to the condition besetting Canada's children as "TV Legs" because lying in front of the TV "decreases flexibility," leads to "posture defects," "obesity" and health risks associated with the tension built up when there is emotional stimulation without adequate physical outlet. This struck a nerve in those of the older generation who were already distrustful of television and its influence on the young and helped the phrase "TV Legs" gain a life of its own.

In Toronto, *The Don Mills Study* and "TV Legs" were front page news and were discussed in a page six editorial. North York politicians used the results of the study as the starting point for a debate on the need to clear sidewalks in winter, and New Democratic Party Member of Parliament, Dan Brown, introduced Percival's findings to the House of Commons as a challenge to the Liberal government's record on promoting physical fitness. Percival was in great demand and made at least two appearances on CBC current affairs programs – radio of course – where he discussed the *Don Mills Mass*

Study as well as adult fitness and offered some insights into his own road to personal fitness. He told listeners that the point was not just to add "years to your life, but more importantly, to add life to your years" and even made reference to "Casanova and the great lovers in history" as products of their physical activities such as fencing. Relating sex to fitness was nothing new for Percival. That favourite slogan of his about physical fitness making "the sky bluer" often included the phrase "even the sex is better" when it was appropriate to the audience he was addressing. Newspaper columnists appreciated Percival's candour on the subject and sometimes elicited his opinions regarding sex and a healthy marriage. On one occasion his forthrightness got him into a great deal of trouble.

In May of 1958, a story emerged regarding a teenage "sex club" in Don Mills. The press took great interest in the incident and managed to associate it with the new North American suburban phenomenon known as "key clubs," where adults swapped partners through an exchange of keys. As Chairman of the Community Association, Percival was asked to comment on the story. His open attitude towards the subject of sex and typically frank comments led to some confusion regarding his response as well as to his attitude towards teenage sex. A few people came to his defence and said that he had been misquoted, but others in the Community Association as well as a large contingent from with the community were outraged, and Percival had to spend much of the next Association meeting convincing the membership that he should not be impeached. As he stated to a *Globe and Mail* reporter, "My reputation has been completely assassinated in Don Mills. I could certainly never run as Mayor." As Joe Taylor says, "Lloyd would fall into controversy the way some people get out of bed."

Fitness for Your Children was Percival's comprehensive response to the findings of the *Don Mills Mass Study*. It was dedicated to assisting parents in raising fit, healthy children. Percival argued that this was of paramount importance to Canadian society because, unlike their parents who were losing a basic level of fitness that most had gained naturally through childhood, this generation of children was threatened with never attaining a sufficient level of fitness and therefore:

> Will not be able to participate adequately in physical activities, will have less energy, be more accident prone, be more likely to develop emotional and mental health problems and will likely become a physically sub-par adult who will probably produce sub-par children.

It was Percival's contention that the physical fitness of children should be treated in the same manner as "regular medical examinations, dental hygiene, nutrition, and other factors involved in healthy, happy living."

The opening argument in the final volume of the four major "Sports College" publications, *How to Stay Slim and Healthy*, could just as easily be delivered today:

> Medical research provides more and more convincing proof every day that excess weight is one of the great enemies of physical fitness, good health and long life. Yet, despite the widening bombardment of publicity this fact now receives, study indicates that more Canadians are becoming overweight every day.

> This alarming trend is not confined to adults. It includes our youth as well. This we discovered when we compared the incidence of excess poundage among teenagers in 1956 with that we had noted during studies made in 1950. The increase was 15 percent.

While we have learned the efficacy of what seemed like odd ideas at the time and have embraced many of Percival's pronouncements on the relationship between nutrition and health, western society has yet to learn the founding principle or "The Key to Weight Control" as he called it in this publication. This is the remarkably simple concept of balance: "People become too fat or too thin – but mostly too fat – because they do not eat according to their actual needs." It is typical of Percival that he believed that people did not understand this concept because they had not been given the knowledge. In this book he provided all of the information necessary to develop not just a balanced diet, but a diet balancing caloric needs against energy consumption. Simply put, in order to maintain a constant weight, the calories a person ingests in a day must equal the calories he or she burns off in a day. To assist his readers, Percival presented a chart of sixty-five daily activities from sleeping to office work to playing football and assigned a value in calories per hour burned for each activity. Percival estimated the daily caloric usage of an average sedentary man to be 2,315.

Other charts attached caloric values to more than five hundred food items. During any twenty-four hour period, Percival's "average sedentary man" had to consume items on this chart that totalled no more than 2,315 calories, or he would gain weight. Obviously an athlete could, and should, consume more calories, but the formula remained the same. Even an athlete will gain weight if he or she consumes more calories than he or she burns off. The concept is so straightforward that Percival subtitled the book *the sure way to solve your weight problems once and for all*. It is so simple that one wonders why it was absent from diet plans in Percival's time and, sadly, why it is so rarely found in diet regimens today.

Some of the most respected coaches in the United States were known to consult with Percival and subscribe to these "Sports College" publications. Football coaches showed a particularly strong interest and included some of the most innovative and successful coaches in the history of the sport: University of Oklahoma coach, Bud Wilkinson; Paul Brown of the NFL Cleveland Browns; Don Shula of the Baltimore Colts; and the Miami Dolphins and San Diego Charger's coach, Sid Gillman. Another Hall of Fame football coach, George Allan, was an assistant with the Chicago Bears in the early 1960s. When a fire destroyed the team offices, Allan sent Percival an urgent request to replenish the Bear's library of coaching textbooks.

In Canada, "Sports College" and its publications were the primary source of information on health, fitness and exercise for an entire generation. Beginning in 1948, the budget for "Sports College" was over $50,000 per year and estimates of the value of the network time, provided free by the CBC, ranged from $100,000 to $150,000 per year. The Physical Fitness Division of the Department of National Health and Welfare, which had been created by the National Physical Fitness Act of 1944, had a budget of only $54,004.15 in 1947-1948 along with $89,635.29 that it was supposed to distribute to the provinces. "Sports College" spent more money informing Canadian youth about sport and a healthy lifestyle than did the federal government and distributed twice as much printed material. When the National Physical Fitness Act was repealed in 1954, government initiatives became even more impotent and, for the rest of the decade, Percival and "Sports College" – the radio broadcasts and the publications – were virtually alone in informing Canadians about health, fitness and how to develop athletic ability.

As a result of the financial demands of maintaining "Sports College" and his frustration with the federal government's continued disinterest in funding fitness initiatives, Percival gave birth to sports marketing in Canada. A key moment came when a request from Moscow for information regarding "Sports College" programming for training and motivating young people made him realize that he wasn't doing enough; that "it was about time we got to work here in Canada on a plan for our own boys and girls." An ambitious program was fully evolved in Percival's ever active imagination by the fall of 1956 when he announced negotiations for funding were progressing with a prominent business concern. It took Percival more than two years, but in the spring of 1959 the "Sports College Junior Champs Club" was unveiled with Nabisco Foods Limited as the sponsor. Percival told the *Globe and Mail*: "The Government does not seem interested in any kind of national fitness scheme, so business and industry is the answer."

Membership in the Junior Champs Club was free to all youths, male and female, who filled out a membership form and attempted a simple home fitness test. Each member received a membership card signed by Lloyd Percival, Head Coach, and Mr. Muscles (Doug MacLennan), Head Trainer, a club crest and a catalogue of available merchandise and literature. Along with one Shredded Wheat box top, a club t-shirt cost $1.00 and a baseball glove was $5.49. Also available were a baseball tips movie, a "How to be a Champ" 45 rpm record of Percival's coaching tips and a set of barbells. The barbells must have raised a few eyebrows because Percival was advocating, and providing instructions for, a safe weightlifting program for youths at least ten years before professional sports advocated it for adults. Members were given incentives to improve their levels of fitness. If their test scores rose to a certain level they earned a "Canadian Champion" crest; at an even higher level they received an "All Star Trophy."

Percival reported that Nabisco Foods Limited was spending $200,000 to underwrite the program in the first year. In return, they received advertising space on all of the literature and on "Sports College" publications. Nabisco used the opportunity to identify the company with healthy eating and the strong family values promoted by "Sports College." Since the special purchases required the submission of one box top, this was one of Percival's most commercial endeavours and probably the first Canadian example of a fully evolved marketing campaign for sport and fitness. It was definitely the first that was both national and bilingual.

The *Sports College Research Guide (SCRG)* and its successor, the *Sports College News (SCN)*, were also used by Percival as a marketing tool through the Product Research division of "Sports College" that was introduced in the first issue of the *SCRG*. Percival's use of product research became a vital cog in the continued development of "Sports College" as well as a lightning rod for criticism directed at him. While he claimed to be responding to a problem "Sports College" had experienced in answering enquiries such as "what is the best type of sports equipment?" and "should an athlete drink soft drinks?" it is obvious that the long articles devoted to research on certain products were commercially driven and that the manufacturers of these products paid for advertising in the *SCRG*. This prompted Percival's critics to accuse him of abandoning the ideals of amateurism and to complain that he was getting rich off of his enterprises.

In Percival's defence, most of the companies that paid for advertising space and found their products receiving positive reviews from the research department – products such as Vaseline, Olympene liniment, Brex High Fibre cereal, Royal Jelly, tea and honey – fit comfortably within the "Sports College" mandate and some contributed to the public education on health and fitness in which Percival was constantly engaged. One of Percival's first sponsors was the Tea Council of Canada which produced a handsome brochure titled, *The Origins of Sport and the Part Tea Plays*. The brochure contained fifteen pages of excellent background information on various sports, a small space devoted to promoting tea, an introduction to Percival and "Sports College" and the recipe for Percival's "Tea Jack-Up."

There were other products such as Sweet Marie chocolate bars, Crush Beverages, Philishave electric shavers and the Continental Casualty Insurance Company that were not in the business of promoting health and well-being. While he did subject these products to some research and did not seem dishonest in the infomercials he created, Percival's promotion of these products was done just for the money and his actions can most kindly be described as pragmatic. Percival's relationship with Crush Beverages is an excellent example of how he dealt with this type of product.

Crush was a major sponsor of "Sports College" for more than a decade, and his association with the soft drink manufacturer invited controversy at the 1954 British Empire Games. While he offered his "Sports College" seal of approval to a product that was certainly not part of an athlete's ideal diet, and Crush would run full page ads in the *Toronto Telegram* associating Crush beverages with a healthy lifestyle along with the claim that theirs was "The ONLY soft drink recommended by Sports College," Percival had ascertained that the beverage was not harmful and did indeed contain some "natural orange juice." Unlike some training experts who banned all soft drinks, Percival offered practical advice on how to enjoy a moderate intake of Crush soft drinks while maintaining a proper athletic diet. In 1953, Percival worked with Crush to publish an informative little booklet titled *How to be Physically Fit* by Lloyd Percival. In return for their logo being prominently featured on the cover, Crush paid to print the booklet and mailed one out, free of charge, to anyone who submitted a request.

Percival never thought that the compromises he made in order to finance his operations diminished his credibility. It is doubtful he would have even called them compromises. Percival was adamant that he control everything and none of his sponsors had any input into programming or publications. As for Percival getting rich from these endorsements, nothing could be further from the truth. In most cases, the money provided by sponsors barely supported the promotion of health and fitness inherent in the programs associated with them. When there was money left over it was used to maintain the numerous, non-revenue producing "Sports College" activities. If Percival had wanted to become rich he had plenty of opportunities, and none included operating "Sports College" for $4,000.00 per year – including expenses. Percival originated sport marketing in Canada not because he saw it as a way of making money, but because he was the first person in Canada to understand that the positive image of sport and fitness activities could be bartered with the corporate world in return for the funds needed to promote health and fitness in Canada.

The Canadian Amateur Sport and Fitness Development Service

In 1956, Percival's frustration with the federal government's disinterest in promoting health and fitness for Canadians and his recognition that corporate sponsorship was the way of the future inspired the creation of the Canadian Amateur Sports and Physical Fitness Development Service (CASPFDS). The core of CASPFDS was to be "Sports College of the Air" along with a "Sports College" television program produced independently of the CBC by Joel Aldred's Fifeshire Films and then syndicated. Canoeist Bert Oldershaw, who had trained with Percival for the 1952 Olympics and who was preparing for his third Olympics that summer, was named Chairman of a National Advisory Council that would include representatives from sport, physical and health education, recreation, medicine and the media. CASPFDS was intended to increase participation in sport and recreation, build facilities, develop coaches, improve public awareness and provide top level competition. The ultimate goal was "to make Canadians the most amateur sports and fitness conscious and knowledgeable people in the world."

Through private enterprise, Percival was attempting to create what other countries were building through government directed and sponsored programs, and nothing like it would actually come to fruition in Canada until the twenty-first century. In spite of the big numbers Percival loved to boast of in relation to "Sports College," everything he had ever done paled beside this enterprise, and therein lay the major flaw. This was not something he could build or run on his own. The success of CASPFDS would depend upon the voluntary support of sports and fitness individuals and groups throughout Canada as well as on private fundraising for an annual budget of $700,000. Percival stated that he was going ahead with the project because he had been convinced through conversations with people all across Canada that both the human and financial supports were available. He was wrong. With only three television stations

in Canada not affiliated with the CBC and no history of syndica-
tion, the television program died. Fundraising at this level was not
feasible at the time and the level of co-operation amongst the various interest groups was impossible especially with a polarizing figure
such as Percival at the helm.

The failure of CASPFDS does not alter the fact that it was
inspired and revolutionary. Had Percival succeeded, Canada would
have become a world leader in fitness and amateur sport; however,
he was speaking a different language from those around him and, as
was often the fate with his programs, CASPFDS was so far ahead of
its time that failure was inevitable. More than a decade later, when
the federal government established Sports Canada, people would
begin to understand Percival's language, but it would not be until
2004 when *Own the Podium 2010* was established that the language
became clear. As brilliant as the concept was, this was one of the few
times in his life when Percival completely misjudged the situation
and vastly overestimated his abilities.

Undeterred by the failure of CASPFDS, Percival and "Sports
College" carried on as usual. Two more research papers were published, each demonstrating how the poor fitness levels of Canadians
were both avoidable and reversible. One was a tightly controlled
study of 109 adults (seventy-nine males and thirty females) with
an average age of thirty-eight (age range twenty-six to forty-nine).
All of the subjects were considered sedentary – that is – "none had
participated in regular exercise of any kind for an average of seven
years, 72 had been physically active in youth, 37 had been relatively
inactive in youth." Percival wrote, "as far as we can ascertain this is
the first study ever conducted designed specifically to actually check
what does happen when sedentary adults sustain a program of progressive exercise over a period of at least six months."

Typical of Percival was the inclusion of subjective questions
regarding tension, emotional well-being, ability to sustain mental
effort, feelings of general health and satisfaction with sexual capacity. As pleased as he was that the results of his study demonstrated

that an unfit Canadian adult, at the stage of life that was then considered middle-aged, could dramatically improve his or her heart fitness, flexibility, strength and posture through regular exercise, it was more important to him that the participants reported a significant improvement in their mental, emotional and sexual well-being.

The second paper was actually a *Maclean's* article, published on March 14, 1959, written by Percival with the help of Trent Frayne on the efforts of "a flabby man in his forties" ... "a typical middle-aged man" named Lloyd Percival to regain his "physical health." Percival had retired from competitive cricket in 1946. By 1954, his weight had ballooned to 181 pounds, 35 pounds above his playing weight. The *Maclean's* article describes in detail Percival's five year ordeal so that the average person could understand that it may seem daunting, but it was possible for an unfit middle-aged Canadian to become fit and, most importantly, that it was worth it.

Percival stressed in the magazine that one did not need five years to accomplish this. He claimed that he had built tests within his test in order to better understand the process and had thereby dragged out the proceedings in the interest of research. With the kind of fitness programs available through "Sports College," the transformation could be relatively simple he advised. At the end of it all, Percival weighed 158 pounds, was much more muscular than before and was just "three pounds over leanness," was able to run twelve miles and could do 159 push-ups in a session. This was the fitness profile that was available to all middle-aged Canadians. Percival would not continue his running regimen but did continue with a limited daily exercise program for the rest of his life. Although, due to his chain smoking and short, barrel-chested physique, he did not appear to be very fit.

Percival summed up his work in the 1940s and 1950s in a "Sports College" publication titled *A Report on the Fitness of Canadians*:

> In its attempt to awaken Canadians to the need for
> fitness activity and the dangers of low fitness levels,

> Sports College conducted over 1,000 national
> radio broadcasts, 44 national newspaper releases,
> prepared 11 articles for national magazines, gave
> 194 speeches, conducted 47 clinics, published 19
> booklets, bulletins and pamphlets of which 900,000
> were distributed, appeared on 7 TV feature
> interviews, produced and distributed two films
> devoted to fitness education, dealt with thousands
> of letters asking for specific information and
> distributed over 1,000,000 catalogues describing
> material Canadians could get to improve fitness
> and exhorting them to start a fitness program.
> Over 200,000 requests for information alone were
> received as a result of the C.B.C. radio program.

This impressive list helps us appreciate the tremendous influence Percival exerted on Canadian society following WWII and how "Sports College" was the heart and soul of his efforts. The benefits accrued by the CBC continued to justify their investment in the program; however, some of Percival's controversial positions, especially regarding nutrition, brought criticism on Canada's national radio network. On one broadcast Percival advised listeners to give up animal fats and use vegetable oils instead. The CBC received numerous letters criticizing the advice and questioning Percival's qualifications regarding nutrition and health. Executives at the network contacted the Food and Drug Directorate of the National Department of Health in Ottawa which, after consulting with a number of "eminent nutritionists" in the United States, advised that:

> Evidence is lacking in medical research for changes
> in physical fitness related to the type of dietary fat.
> … Authorities have recommended no change in
> the general food patterns in view of insufficient
> knowledge to warrant revised food habits with
> respect to fat.

Percival was directed to cease his warnings against animal fat and was asked to provide his supervisors with details of his sources whenever he discussed medical and nutritional matters. Percival was not a nutritionist nor did he come up with these ideas on his own. He read constantly and kept himself up to date on everything related to health, fitness and sport, and even those closest to him were constantly amazed by his encyclopaedic knowledge on just about everything. His voracious appetite for knowledge, combined with what close associates called a "photographic memory," was crucial to his ability to disseminate such an incredible amount of information during the twenty-one years of "Sports College." What is equally important, however, was his critical judgment. New and revolutionary ideas on nutrition and fitness were commonplace in the late 1950s. Just as so many turn out to be worthless today, expensive and useless shortcuts to fitness and health were regularly publicized in Percival's day. Percival always checked his sources and usually conducted his own research. Time has validated most of the products and ideas he endorsed.

Bill C-131: The Fitness and Amateur Sport Act

With a new decade on the horizon, the Conservative government in Ottawa finally began to look seriously at funding fitness and amateur sport and filling the void left when the Liberals repealed the NPFA in 1955. World politics, the Canadian economy and the Royal family all played a part, but the effects of a decade of hectoring by Lloyd Percival cannot be discounted.

This was the Cold War era. The Russians had just launched Sputnik and North Americans were still building bomb shelters. In less than a decade, athletes from the Soviet Union had become the dominant force in amateur sport, and the world had witnessed a politicization of sport far beyond the scope Percival had experienced in Berlin in 1936. Percival often quoted from Kipling:

Nations have passed away and left no traces
And history gives the naked cause of it -
One single, simple reason in all cases:
They fell because their peoples were not fit!

He cautioned that Western Civilization was going the way of the Romans because it was becoming "passive" and "sedentary" and dependent on "automation. ... these days we have a car in every garage to keep us sedentary. The ancients who grew soft had a chariot in every courtyard." Percival shared societies' concern over the space race but advised Canadians that they were losing another equally important competition with the Eastern Bloc countries:

Little concern has been shown about the fact that
the Russians and other Communist-dominated
countries are even further ahead in their work with
probably the most important machine of all – the
human body. The Communists have been quick to
realize the role which fitness can play in building
work-energy, morale and physical and emotional
stamina. These things are the very essence of
vitality and enthusiasm; of the ability to endure
and thus can be classified as extremely important
prerequisites of any long term war (cold or hot).

The Cold War era was one of fear, but it was also one of prosperity for Canada's growing urban middle class. It provided more taxes for the government to work with and evolved a more relaxed attitude toward government sponsored health and fitness activities. This growing middle class also spent a great deal of time in front of those new televisions. Since much of this time was spent watching sports, they became increasingly aware of how poorly Canadian athletes were faring in international competition. Politicians sensed a general dissatisfaction with Canada's international athletes – especially the hockey teams – as well as a desire to see something done about it.

It is generally accepted that a much publicized speech by the Duke of Edinburgh, Prince Phillip, to the Canadian Medical Association in June of 1959 in which he lamented the poor state of physical fitness in Canada and challenged the medical profession to do something about it prompted the government to finally take action. Historians, however, also point to efforts during the 1950s of Ian Eisenhardt, leader of British Columbia's Pro-Rec movement; Doris Plewes, physical fitness consultant for the federal Ministry of Health and Welfare; and Lloyd Percival, going so far as to state that Prince Phillip simply "echoed fitness radio personality Lloyd Percival's frequent fitness messages on his show, *Sports College of the Air.*"

Prime Minister John Diefenbaker's visit to the Pan American Games in Chicago in 1960 provided further impetus. In a November 1960 speech to the House of Commons, Diefenbaker proclaimed:

> In the field of sports today there are tremendous dividends in national pride from some degree of success in athletics. The uncommitted countries of the world are now using these athletic contests as measurements of the evidence of the strength and power of the nations participating.

Behind the scenes, Douglas Fisher and J.W. Willard were instrumental in driving the sport and fitness agenda forward. Fisher never forgot his conversation with Lloyd Percival in 1953, and the promotion of sport was one of his main objectives after he was elected as the CCF – the precursor of the NDP – Member for Port Arthur, Ontario, in 1957. Willard became Deputy Minister of Health in 1960 and Fisher credits him with immediately changing the climate in the ministry, thereby enabling the voices of the sports and fitness lobbyists to be heard.

On September 25, 1961, Bill C-131, the *Fitness and Amateur Sport Act*, was passed with unanimous consent. Its stated purpose was "to encourage, promote and develop fitness and amateur sport in Canada." The Act represented a major turning point in government policy:

> For the first time, government was committed
> to the promotion and development of amateur
> sport and not just to general physical fitness. They
> demonstrated their commitment in monetary
> terms: A maximum of $1,000,000 would be
> allocated the first year. That figure would rise
> by $1,000,000 each year until it levelled off at an
> annual commitment of $5,000,000 per year.

One week before the final reading of the bill, Minister of Health and Welfare Hon. J.W. Monteith had introduced the measure in a speech delivered to Parliament. The speech was written by Douglas Fisher. In that speech, Monteith paid homage to Percival and the others who had been fighting so long for this legislation:

> These and others have been outspoken champions
> of fitness and amateur sport, and have repeatedly
> urged some form of assistance from the Dominion
> Government in support of such activities. While
> it has not been possible to implement all of their
> specific arguments, I hope that they will find in our
> new proposals the achievement of at least the spirit
> of their intention.

A Phoenix Rises in Don Mills

A**S MUCH AS THE TRACK AND FIELD COMMUNITY WISHED IT**, Percival had never really gone away. He served as an advisor to Joe Taylor until the last of the Red Devils moved on at the end of 1954 and assisted Taylor and Paul Poce at Toronto Olympic Club in 1955. He avoided responding to Jackie MacDonald's requests for help preparing her for the 1955 Pan American Games in Mexico and the 1956 Olympics but was quite happy to refer to himself as MacDonald's coach in feature stories on the young prodigy that appeared in the *Toronto Star* and in *Maclean's* April, 1955. He was regularly asked for his opinions on track and field matters by sportswriters such as Bobbi Rosenfeld who questioned the integrity and judgement of Canadian track and field officials when they failed to invite Percival to coaching seminars they were sponsoring. In June 1955, Rosenfeld repeated Percival's call for an overall "recruiting, training and coaching plan" for Canadian track and field and introduced a fifteen article series penned by Percival and titled "Olympic Hints." It was, in effect, a set of "Sports College" mini-training manuals offered free to anyone who read the newspaper and, as a unit, comprised a track and field training program that was as good as anything published at that time.

Fred Foot was named Head Track and Field coach for the 1956 Olympic Games in large part because five of the seventeen Canadian track and field athletes headed for Melbourne came from his East York club. Two of the five, however, were Percival's protégés (MacDonald and Murray Cockburn). Another former Red Devil, Shirley Eckel (Kerr), believes that she was left off of the team due to her past association with Percival. Eckel had not joined East York, preferring to train on her own. Running in four inches of sludge in the inside lane of a water-logged cinders track, Eckel failed to meet the Olympic standard at the Canadian trials; however, she had run under the qualifying standard in her eighty metre hurdles event at a sanctioned meet in the United States shortly before the Canadian trials (she had also finished second at the USA National Championships), and before Foot went into the selection meeting, Eckel presented him with a sworn statement from the American meet director verifying that she had run the required time. When the team was announced, Eckel's name was not on the list. She was used to the whims of the badgers, had no coach to stand up for her and did not protest. It was only later that she learned that Foot had failed to produce her letter at the meeting and did not make a case for her to be named to the team. Canada did not have an entry in the women's eighty metre hurdles in Melbourne. For the second time, Shirley Eckel missed out on an opportunity to represent her country in the Olympics and, for the second time, Canada was denied one of its best opportunities for a medal in track and field.

The team that Canada sent to Melbourne was very small and, as usual, short of funds. Percival did his best to raise money, helping Foot organize an exhibition mile with "Olympic contenders" during half-time at a Toronto Argonaut football game. He also spoke out in the press over the size of the budget the COA had to work with ($216,900, if they managed to raise that much). Percival compared it to the amount of money the Canadian government had given to long-distance swimmers since 1954 ($178,200) and wondered about the country's priorities. Canadians won six medals in Melbourne, three more than in Helsinki; however, the improvement was attributable to one man, Frank Read, the exceptional coach of the University of British Columbia (UBC) rowing team. Track and field athletes again failed to win even one medal and Percival continued to criticize track and field officials at every opportunity. He did not stop there. In 1959, Percival wrote an article for *Ontario Today Magazine* in which he stated, "As far as coaching is concerned, most Canadian coaches are actually still twenty-five years behind the times with few exceptions."

It was Percival's love of working with young people that finally caused him to stop criticizing from the sidelines and return to coaching track and field. His involvement with his new Don Mills community led to a fitness/track and field program at the local Y.M.C.A. It did not start as a competitive club. There were only "field days" organized by the Y.M.C.A., and Percival seemed content to introduce the eight to twelve year olds to the joys of track and field. Within a couple of years, however, the joy of competition Percival witnessed in these children brought him back to the glory and the pettiness of competitive track and field – opposite points of the compass that brought out both the best and the worst in him.

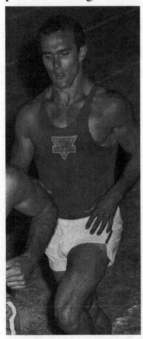

Bill Gairdner competing in a 400 meter heat for a decathlon competition in 1962.

In co-operation with the Don Mills Y.M.C.A., Percival began an "experimental" track and field program in 1958 involving seventy-eight children aged six to fourteen along with two older teenagers,

Bill Gairdner and Bob Meldrum. Seven of the youngsters entered the Ontario age class championships in September of that year and brought home "two firsts, four seconds and four thirds" even though they were generally younger than their competition. In 1959, Percival took the Don Mills Y Track Club to meets in London and Montreal. Soon, John Hudson, captain of the track team at Dubuque University and future National Track and Field coach, joined the Don Mills group as an assistant, and Percival was set for another assault on Canadian track and field records as well as on the sensibilities of track and field officials.

Percival didn't waste any time before letting the badgers know that he was back. On the eve of the 1960 Olympics in Rome, he had a conversation with Gabrial Korobkov, a top-level Russian track and field coach, who was leading a Russian track team on a tour of the United States. Korobkov asked Percival why Canadian hockey players were "strong, fast and brave," but Canadians "were not progressing in track and field?" Percival told Korobkov that Canada had "many excellent young prospects" but that most could not afford to attend the national trials "at which there were just about as many officials as athletes." Percival turned his meeting with Korobkov into a three page press release on the problems besetting track and field in Canada and took dead aim at the badgers: "We have very little to show for the past few years except a few aging veteran officials whose progress can be measured only in miles traveled."

By the summer of 1960, the Don Mills Y Track Club was a powerful force, and Percival was once again attempting to change the culture of track and field in Canada. The Don Mills Y.M.C.A. had to abandon sole sponsorship of the club when the budget exceeded their resources, but the Don Mills Track Club would always remain a community project. Although there were still only five very young women on the team, Don Mills won the Women's Title at the Ontario Senior Track and Field Championships in London in 1960. The women's team continued to grow and the great success Percival had enjoyed coaching female athletes in the early 1950s was surpassed by his female track and field competitors of the 1960s. The feminist movement of the late 1960s would be a turning point for women in sport, but there were still many myths regarding menstruation, pregnancy and motherhood, and the ability of women to withstand exertion for any length of time was still in question. The success of the Eastern European women in dispelling some of these myths was undermined by questions regarding their femininity, but Percival insisted that "the sportswoman is now the ultimate in femininity." He not only advocated for the competitive athletic aspirations of women, he asserted, "Canadian women have much greater athletic potential then the men. They're fitter and more dedicated."

In spite of the youth and inexperience around him, Percival took on the task of organizing the Olympic Decathlon Trials set for July 9th and 10th, 1960, at Don Mills Collegiate. It became a Don Mills community project, and Percival boasted that everything would be "state of the art" and up to Olympic standards, something "no other track and field event in Canada" could claim. Percival brought in "three of Toronto's leading chartered accountants" to tabulate the results and staged a Miss Decathlon contest to ensure better media coverage. The meet was first-class, and Percival earned rare plaudits from the Chairman of the Central Ontario Committee of the AAU, Dick Harding.

The 1960 Olympic Games were an unmitigated disaster for Canada. Canada's only medal was won by Frank Read's UBC rowers who, in spite of the glory they had brought to Canada four years earlier, had been reduced to carrying tin cups around Empire Stadium during BC Lions football games gathering donations prior to the Games. None of the rising stars in the Don Mills club were ready for international competition, and it was no surprise that the club was not represented on the 1960 Olympic team; however, Percival did make some contribution to whatever talent Canada did send to Rome. Jim Mossman, coach of the canoeing team, recalls waiting at Toronto's Malton Airport (precursor to the Pearson International Airport) with the rest of the Canadian delegation bound for Rome.

When Percival unexpectantly arrived to see the athletes off, Mossman was surprised to find that almost half of the Canadian athletes seemed to have personal relationships with Percival.

In spite of the dismal showing in Rome the future looked bright not only for Percival's young charges, but also for a new generation of track and field athletes in Ontario. The absolute domination of the Toronto Track and Field Club between 1946 and 1954 had been due as much to the sheer incompetence of the other coaches as it was to Percival's brilliance. By 1960, there were many good coaches running strong track and field programs in Ontario, notably two whose careers were born of the seminal period of the early 1950s – Fred Foot, who did double duty with East York Track Club and the University of Toronto Track Club, and Paul Poce with the Toronto Olympic Club. Even high school athletes now received quality coaching from the likes of future University of Toronto and national team coach, Andy Higgins who "grew up listening to Sports College and 'devoured' all of the Sports College publications he could get his hands on," and former Red Devil, Murray Gaziuk. These coaches were also producing national and international calibre athletes, and they deserved respect. All too often Percival's ego kept him from acknowledging their expertise. In 1963, Irish coach, Geoff Dyson, was hired to conduct the first in a series of annual coaching clinics in Guelph. He brought with him from the British Isles a number of excellent coaches including Peter Radford, Lionel Pugh and Geoff Gowan, who all later became national team coaches and administrators in Canada. Percival was invited to take part but declined. He told John Hudson, "they only want me there to give them credibility." Percival was angry because he had wanted to organize such clinics for years but no one would listen to him. When he was invited as a participant, he took it as an insult. Percival was never good at being a participant. He only wanted to lead.

Although Percival and his precocious troop did a great deal to raise the profile of track and field in Canada during this time and helped attract young people into the sport, they were field event competitors for the most part, and their specialties were not likely to grab the attention of the public. It was two young men from Fred Foot's East York club who heralded the dawning of this Golden Age of track and field in Canada. Bruce Kidd and Bill Crothers were competitors in the high profile middle distance events and became stars on the American indoor circuit which was blossoming into a major television attraction. This translated into greater media interest in Canada and meant that track and field was no longer as dependant on Percival's skills as a publicist. As veteran sportswriter Al Sokol wrote, "he (Percival) was great for track because he got it in the news. It was a very low profile sport until Bruce Kidd came along."

John Hudson, Fred Foot and Ken Twigg, chairman of the AAU track and field committee, banked on the new found enthusiasm for track and field when they organized the Toronto Telegram - Maple Leaf Indoor Games on January 25, 1963. World class American athletes came north to compete against the new Canadian heroes, and 12,625 paid to see track and field in Maple Leaf Gardens for the first time in twenty-seven years. They did not go home disappointed. Percival's newest young phenom, Nancy McCredie, started things off by smashing the Canadian record for the shot put, Bruce Kidd broke the Canadian three mile record, Crothers defeated his American rivals and the evening ended with a world record in the pole vault.

Twigg then teamed up with Percival to stage the Toronto International Games outdoors at Varsity Stadium on June 25th. With world class competitors recruited from the United States and the great young Canadian talent, Percival said it would be "the finest meet ever held in the country." That summer Bill Gairdner of the Don Mills club finished third in the decathlon at the Pan American Games, becoming the first Canadian to win a decathlon medal in international competition. Gairdner acknowledges that he owes much of his success to Percival's coaching and his "kinaesthetic imagination," an innate ability Percival had honed through years of study and work with athletes. It was the main reason that he was a fine athletic trainer and was a key factor in so many of the Don Mills athletes becoming Canadian champions. With the 1964 Olympics just around the corner, Ontario had supplanted British Columbia as the hotbed of track and field in Canada, and Canada's prospects for the Tokyo Olympics looked better than they had since the 1920s.

In 1964, the Don Mills Club was again scheduled to host the Canadian Decathlon/Pentathlon Trials. Suddenly, a little over one month prior to the July 30th event, Percival announced their withdrawal citing COTFA president Desmond Bellew's insistence on eliminating three races and all of the field events from the schedule. Percival had introduced these events in order to fill the time while pentathletes and decathletes recovered between events, as well as to entertain the crowd during the delays. He defended this program with references to his successful 1960 meet, as well as to similar American and European meets, and insisted that his main concern was the health and well-being of the decathletes. Percival knew more about organizing a decathlon/pentathlon meet than did Bellew; however, it's possible he could have made compromises to satisfy the COFTA president – Percival claimed that he was never given that opportunity. Instead, this looks like an example of Percival's refusal to compromise, his tendency to publicly denounce his adversaries and to walk away if they failed to acknowledge that he was in the right. In the end, it didn't matter who was in the right. The conflict exacerbated Percival's perpetually strained relationship with the rest of the track and field community.

Bill Crothers was particularly incensed by Percival's decision and made his feelings known in a letter to Percival, written on official East York Track Club stationary. Crothers was already a star in Canadian track and field and had established a squeaky clean image within and without the track and field community. In the years since, he has gained a well-deserved reputation as an honest and honourable man; however, this petty and vindictive epistle suggests that Crothers already possessed considerable animosity towards Percival:

Dear Lloyd:

I hope the paper that I am typing on isnit (sic) spoiled, because I have been reading so much concerning your troubles lately that when I read tonight's <u>Star</u>, I burst out crying. Some of my tears might have landed on the paper and soiled it.

Why don't you quit acting like a spoiled, arrogant, self-pitied child. I realize that most of your athletes are only midgets – and for that I respect you – but that is no reason why you have to act about the same age.

This stunt of pulling out of holding the Decathlon and Pentathlon Trials and the publicity that you have made sure resulted from it is pretty ridiculous. It may be your right to decline to hold these Trials if you so choose – but if you do decline, then you must be adult enough to accept the responsibility, and not blame somebody else for your troubles. It is quite obvious that you were not showing too much respect or consideration to the competing athletes who would be at the meet.

Or could the real reason behind your lack of enthusiasm be the fact that Don Mills Track Club athletes no longer are in a position to win either. (Or rather the athletes who are in a position to win are no longer members of the Don Mills Track Club.) I wonder what would have happened if Bill Gairdner was still training in Toronto. If Bob Meldrum and Jenny Wingerson were still with Don Mills. Seems strange that these things seem to be connected.

But then we all know that Lloyd Percival is an honourable man and wouldn't have even considered these happenings, don't we?

Yours truly,
(signature)
Bill Crothers

Crothers defends this letter as the product of a naïve and earnest young man, prone to sarcasm. He claims that he hardly knew Percival at that time and had no personal vendetta against him but resented the negative press Percival generated through this kind of action when the sport had so much trouble gaining publicity at all. Crothers says today that he was simply doing as he always did – standing up for the integrity of the sport.

In October, nine men and six women flew to Japan to represent Canada in track and field at the Olympics. Gairdner was the only male from the Don Mills TC, but three of the six women on the team were coached by Percival: Nancy McCredie, Jenny Wingerson and Marian Snyder. Percival told the press that Canadians should be proud of the great strides that had been made in track and field over the past four years but warned that youth and lack of international experience would present a great challenge to the team; that Canadians should be pleased if the young athletes were able to make the finals and earn points for their country.

Sports College: The Final Years

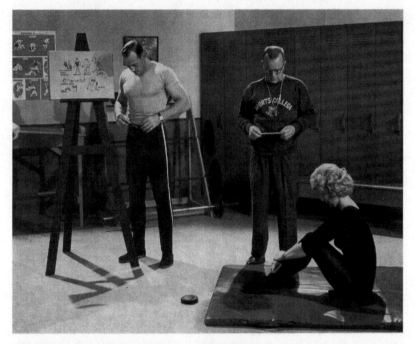

Doug MacLennan, Lloyd Percival and Eileen Boland on the set
of the Sports College television program in 1963.

THE 1960S SAW A NEW GENERATION of executives at the CBC taking a critical look at long-standing programs such as "Sports College." What they found was a radio show that had grown a little tired and lost energy and focus. A succession of young producers made cosmetic changes to the program including a revolving door of announcers – Max Ferguson's long-time sidekick, Alan McPhee, appeared to enjoy his many appearances on "Sports

College," but future ABC News anchorman, Peter Jennings, was less than thrilled to be working on a sports program.

This is not to say that Percival and MacLennan were not still producing informative and even innovative programming. In the December 9, 1961, episode, Percival introduced Cart, "the all stomach short-legs projection of modern man" he predicted would be the fate of Canadians if they failed to change their lifestyle. Personal research along with published medical studies presented by Percival demonstrated that "automatic and labour saving devices" and "passive entertainment" had to be counteracted by regular exercise and healthy eating if Canadians were to get off of the "sedentary slope" they were currently on. This was standard Percival fare; however, the title, a reference to the popular Mel Brooks and Carl Reiner comedy routine, The 2000 Year Old Man, caught the imagination of the public. Cart was widely reported upon at the time, and the segment can be heard today on the CBC Archives internet site.

In spite of Cart and a number of other informative episodes, the radio program was suffering from neglect. Joel Aldred had finally realized his long-time ambition to start a television station when CFTO began broadcasting on December 31, 1961, and Lloyd Percival's "Sports College" was one of the new programs. Percival's television program, also broadcast on independent stations in Winnipeg and Halifax, was based on the format of the radio program. He was enthused about being able to demonstrate exercises, use diagrams, charts and films as well as the short "Facts About Fitness" segments he taped for airing on Friday evenings. But he found it difficult to cope with the constantly changing schedule that started with fifteen minute segments three times a week, was reduced to twice a week and finally became a thirty minute program every Saturday.

The show was cancelled after twenty-one months and had nowhere near the impact of the radio version. Still, many young Canadians in Toronto, Winnipeg and Halifax gained new insights into sports and fitness. Theirs was a new generation that was beginning to learn more from watching then from listening, and Percival understood McLuhan's contention that on television what is said is less important than how it is presented. Doug MacLennan demonstrated all of the exercises and 8 mm films, as well as film clips, were used extensively. When he introduced Mr. 2000 to the television audience, Percival didn't just talk about his "all-stomach short-legs projection of modern man," he presented a puppet version designed by Doug MacLennan.

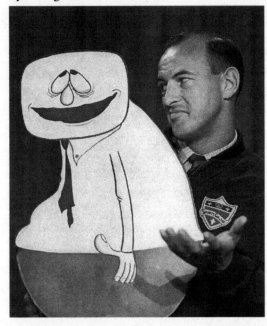

Doug MacLennan holding the puppet figure of "Mr. 2000," used on the Sports College television program on CTV in 1963.

Bill Heikkila was one of the young viewers whose life was changed by the television program. Heikkila was interested in learning to throw the javelin. It is a major sport in Finland, his parents' homeland, but Heikkila had not been able to find a coach in Canada who understood the sport. After seeing films of proper javelin technique on "Sports College" – the television program – one Saturday morning Heikkila joined Percival's Don Mills track club. Percival helped him gain a scholarship to the University of Oregon where he hooked up with another track and field legend, Bill Bowerman. Percival and Bowerman became the "two great mentors" in Heikkila's life and the inspiration for a fine athletic career, surpassed only by thirty-five years of coaching that earned him the City of Ottawa's 2005 "Brian Kilrea Award for Excellence in Coaching."

As well as the television program, Percival was again running the largest track and field club in Canada and was working on plans for a health club. There just weren't enough hours in the day for everything he wanted to do, and MacLennan was occasionally left to do the Saturday radio broadcasts by himself. Percival could never admit that "Sports College of the Air" was suffering. Instead, he expressed shock when on June 4, 1964, he was told that "Sports College" was to be placed on a thirteen week summer hiatus. When Percival protested that he had received no warning and had invested time and money in planning the summer schedule, he was informed that it would be more than a hiatus. "Sports College" was cancelled as of June 27, 1964.

CBC internal memos reveal that certain CBC executives had attempted to terminate "Sports College" as early as 1959, but that longstanding support within the corporation along with other more important program decisions had prevented them from succeeding. By 1964, there were not many CBC executives left who remembered the halcyon days of "Sports College." The young turks in management were anxious to make their mark and introduce their own programming.

Officially, the CBC informed Percival:

> It is our intention to work in the direction of a
> more comprehensive format which will include
> the aims and objectives of many agencies which,
> like your Association, are concerned with physical
> health and education.

Unofficially, the new executives had no interest in producing a program over which they had so little control.

Percival was never one to let someone else dictate terms. He cried foul and argued that the original agreement with the Y.M.C.A., which stipulated a six month notice prior to cancellation, had been accepted by the CBC in 1948 and was still legally binding. When the dispute was finally resolved and a cheque for $3,040.00 was presented to Percival by R.W. McGall, McGall invited the CBC executives at the centre of the dispute to "join me in hoping that all concerned will benefit from this expensive lesson." It is not clear whether the "expensive lesson" referred to the lack of due diligence followed by these executives or to the folly of getting into a fight with Lloyd Percival.

PART III

The Guru 1964–1974

The Fitness Institute

THE HEALTH CLUB PERCIVAL WAS PLANNING would be known as The Fitness Institute. In 1962, Percival had been approached by Eddie Creed, president of Creed's Limited, "Canada's most fashionable fur and dress salon," Murray Koffler, owner of a few Toronto pharmacies that would become the Shoppers Drug Mart chain, and Isadore (Issy) Sharpe of Max Sharpe and Sons, a Toronto construction firm, who were planning a $3,000,000.00 motor hotel on a sixteen acre park setting in North York. In 1961 Creed, Koffler and Sharpe had surprised the established hotel developers with the success of their first hotel, the European style Four Seasons Hotel on Jarvis Street in Toronto. The following year they decided to stretch the boundaries of North American hotel design by introducing "a new concept in hospitality."

When the plans for the Inn on the Park were being finalized, it was discovered that there were 5,000 square feet of space that had not been accounted for. The partners decided to build a health club for hotel guests there. Today, no one would dream of opening a first class hotel without including a state of the art health and fitness facility. In 1963, the concept was fresh and unproven. Creed and Koffler both suggested bringing Lloyd Percival in to equip, staff and operate the health club. Creed knew Percival from his youth in Rosedale; Koffler had become acquainted with Percival through Percival's frequent visits to replenish his trainer's kit at the original Koffler Drug Store in Don Mills. The idea was to ask Percival to install "a typical gym ... a kind of sophisticated Vic Tanny's."

Percival's first reaction was to say that "massaging overweight tourists" did not interest him. The partners persisted. After explaining that this would be his health club, that he could bring his Don Mills Track Club athletes, any Olympic athletes he was assisting and "Sports College" into the facility – as long as the hotel guests were looked after – Percival consulted with Doug MacLennan. MacLennan harboured serious doubts because Percival and MacLennan were already stretched too thin, but Percival had already begun negotiating with wealthy Bay Street Stockbroker, Jim Gairdner, father of Bill Gairdner. When the elder Gairdner agreed to guarantee whatever loans would be required, Percival agreed to the arrangement.

Percival called his new venture The Fitness Institute because it was never intended to be just a health club. It was "a Physical Fitness and Sports Instruction Centre, the first of its kind in the world" where:

> Hotel guests, local residents and industry
> executives may avail themselves of a scientifically
> planned, individually-tailored program designed to
> maintain or shape their physical condition.

Jim Gairdner put up all of the money and took the greatest risk, but Percival told people from day one that Gairdner had promised him a free hand. The Fitness Institute would pay a moderate fee to the Inn on the Park for the space. In return, Percival and his staff would service the recreational and fitness requirements of the hotel guests. Memberships, sold to individuals and businesses in the community, would help defray Gairdner's costs. Percival was to service the needs of the members but was not to worry about turning this into a money making fitness club.

The opening of The Fitness Institute in September 1963 dramatically changed Percival's life. For years he had operated out of cramped offices at the Y.M.C.A., the various downtown spaces he had rented and his Glen Road and Don Mills homes. At The Inn on the Park, there was ample office space for both him and MacLennan as well as reception rooms, and, for the first time, Percival had a fully equipped, onsite gymnasium for training and testing his athletes. In addition to the main exercise room, there were "testing and evaluation rooms, sauna baths (dry and wet steam), a physical treatment room, a locker room, a pro shop, showers, rest facilities and a food bar ... a lecture hall and film area." There was even an "Alpine Board on which mountain climbing (could) be simulated," anticipating the indoor rock climbing craze by forty years. During the summer, members and guests could enjoy the heated outdoor Olympic-style 25 metre swimming pool and a separate diving pool as well as tennis courts and a pitch and putt golf course.

The Fitness Institute did not look like an ordinary health club. It featured the "luxurious appointments of a country club." However, aesthetics were not the only consideration:

> Colour consultants were used to determine the interior and exterior décor. In the testing and evaluation rooms red was chosen for its qualities of sensory stimulation, while in the physical treatment room, colour designs are in soft greens against black to give greater relaxation.

From the opening day, The Fitness Institute employed a full-time receptionist and secretary. Otherwise, like "Sports College," it was still very much a two-man operation. In spite of this, Percival and MacLennan evolved a service model unparalleled at any other North American health club, servicing an ever-growing list of amateur and professional athletes, hotel guests and outside members. Unlike other health clubs of that era, before the male and female members chose from a variety of membership packages, they had to obtain a letter from their doctor declaring them healthy enough to engage in an exercise program, and they filled out an extensive questionnaire regarding their family history, health, fitness and lifestyle. Each new member was then tested and fully evaluated before being presented with a personalized training program. Percival proclaimed it "safe, sure and scientific." Eventually, a Fitness Institute "home" training program was also available to those for whom full membership was not possible. Initially, Percival and MacLennan shared responsibility for developing training programs. Soon, however, Percival was concentrating his efforts on special clients, and MacLennan was largely responsible for the rest.

After producing numerous individual training programs based on Percival's physical training principles, MacLennan noticed that, although each program had its individual variations, there was a great deal of repetition. As membership numbers increased, the time required to assess each member's program and devise individual routines became onerous. He deduced that if clients were grouped according to age, gender and fitness level, standardized programs could be devised that, when adjusted to allow for individual needs, could be produced more quickly and efficiently without compromising the promise of individual attention that was essential to The Fitness Institute service model. MacLennan created a Master Book of exercise programs which he consulted before designing individual programs and which he returned to when revising those programs as he and Percival followed each individual's progress through several levels of fitness. What began as a tool to make life easier for him became one of The Fitness Institute's most important innovations and a way to ensure that each fitness instructor who later joined the staff devised programs that were consistent with the goals of The Fitness Institute and adhered to Percival's methods.

Testing Facilities

The Fitness Institute motto was "Modern Conditioning for the Modern World." With Jim Gairdner's money, Percival acquired whatever equipment that would enable them to fulfill that promise. There was a device that revealed in graphic form the functional fitness of the heart and circulatory system, a Dekan Reaction Timer to measure reaction time and neuro-muscular coordination, a gonioscope for measuring joint and muscle flexibility, a dynamometer for measuring strength, a device to delineate body type and posture defects, a podioscope for determining foot and weight-bearing problems and a heartometer, a very controversial device that some believed helped to evaluate the effects of exercise on the heart. He also purchased the best exercise bicycles and treadmills (which were very hard to find at that time). To anyone with a passing knowledge of exercise equipment this list will appear rudimentary at best; however, in the early 1960s these apparatuses were found only at universities and in hospitals, not in health clubs.

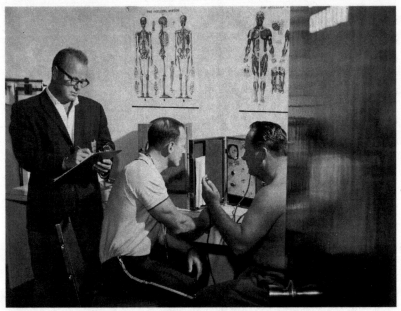

Lloyd Percival (left) in the Inn on the Park Fitness Institute Testing Room with Doug MacLennan (centre) and a Fitness Institute member who is hooked up to a Dekan Reaction Timer.

It wasn't long before Percival could afford to hire a full-time masseur as well as a masseuse for female clients. In the second year, a full-time nurse, Doreen Fraser, joined the staff to supervise fitness testing, and a part-time doctor was consulted regarding member profiles as well as the specific health concerns of some of the members. Finally, a few full-time and part-time fitness instructors, including

Bob Bursach and Lloyd and Dorothy's daughter, Jan, who designed individual programs for the female membership, were hired to help look after the needs of the competitive athletes and the swelling membership list. As long as it was located in The Inn on the Park, however, the success of The Fitness Institute ultimately depended upon the eighty-hour weeks put in by Percival and MacLennan.

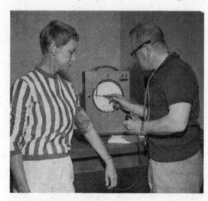

Dorothy Percival at Inn on the Park Fitness Institute and Lloyd Percival checking her fitness with a Heartometer.

The media flocked to The Fitness Institute. It was new and modern in a time when new and modern seemed to be all that mattered, and Percival had a knack for understanding what made for good copy. He gained great mileage out of "Mr. 2000" while aligning himself with recognized authorities such as American heart specialist, Dr. William Raab, who had appeared on his CFTO television program in 1961. In May 1964, the CBC current affairs radio program, "Assignment," featured Percival's commentary on consecutive nights: first as an expert on amateur sport assessing Canada's chances at the upcoming Tokyo Olympics, and the following night as an expert on diet and health issues. In December 1962, columnist Mary Walpole, the doyenne of the Toronto social set, advised her largely female readership that a "year of health and vitality" through membership at The Fitness Institute would be a perfect Christmas gift for their husbands. And Percival was invited to be a judge at a beauty contest that included fitness tests.

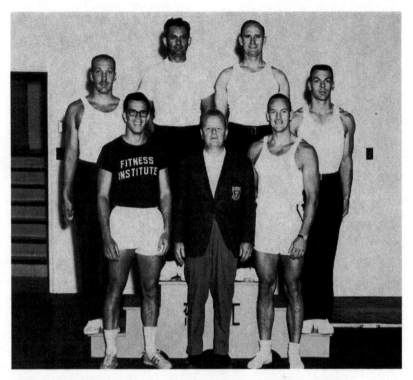

A few of the RCMP trainers visiting The Fitness Institute in 1965 with Lloyd Percival (bottom centre) and Fitness Institute staff member Derek Arbuckle (bottom left), where they were introduced to the new RCMP Physical Training Program Percival had prepared.

At the other end of the spectrum was Canada's law enforcement elite, the Royal Canadian Mounted Police (RCMP), who called on Percival to write a contemporary Canadian replacement for their outdated British-based physical training manual. The three hundred page, two volume *Physical Training and Testing Syllabus* that was introduced to the new RCMP recruits in 1965 allocated significantly more time to physical training than had its predecessor. Much of the new material was standard – at least for Percival; however, just as his sports training programs were always sport specific, this program incorporated the particular physical requirements of an RCMP officer. Percival and MacLennan continued working with senior RCMP staff for more than two years in order to refine the program and feedback from the RCMP instructors charged with implementing the program was enthusiastic.

1964 Tokyo Olympics

A MONGST THE FIRST ATHLETES to make use of the new facilities at The Fitness Institute were the Don Mills Track Club athletes who were seeking berths on the 1964 Olympic team. Marian (Munroe) Snyder was the newest member of the club. From 1957 to 1963 she had been one of the best 60 metre hurdlers in Canada while competing for Fred Foot's East York Track Club. Snyder grew tired of always finishing behind hurdlers from Don Mills and, with her last shot at the Olympics one year away, decided that if she couldn't beat them, she would join the Don Mills club and find out its secret.

When Snyder approached Percival and asked him to train her for the 1964 Olympics, the first thing he told her was that she was training for the wrong event. Having watched her for years, Percival was convinced that Snyder's ideal event was the 800 metres, not the 60 metre hurdles. Since there was not enough time to make such a dramatic change in her training, Percival promised to do his best to prepare her for the hurdles. It didn't take long for Snyder to find out why she had been unable to defeat her Don Mills rivals. The circuit training, testing and indoor training she experienced with Don Mills Track Club, combined with the individual approach to developing training programs, were so far advanced from anything she had been exposed to under Foot that she was sure she would soon be able to challenge Don Mills hurdlers, Jenny Wingerson and Cathy Chapman.

While the intense training made Snyder feel physically and mentally stronger, her hurdling was not improving and her times were not what she and Percival anticipated. What happened next establishes, without a doubt, that Percival was without peer in

Canadian athletic coaching. Even today when an athlete fails to improve, a coach is apt to question the dedication or the innate ability of the athlete, maybe even the intensity of the training regimen, but rarely the coach's own methods. Percival, however, was willing and able to evaluate everything that contributed to athletic performance in order to help his athletes, and a battery of cognitive tests at The Fitness Institute convinced Percival that his coaching methods were the root of Snyder's problem. In more recent years, Snyder has learned that she is slightly dyslexic. While this was not a recognized diagnosis in 1963 the test results helped Percival understand that explaining hurdling technique to Snyder was ineffective. She required a more visual and physical approach to learning. She needed to see and physically feel the required movements and to have drills designed that maximized repetition. This was not an isolated event in Percival's coaching career. In 1951, he had advised the Detroit Red Wings that some hockey players required this kind of approach, and he had employed it with other track and field athletes including hurdler Shirley Eckels who was told to "feel like a swan." Within a week of implementing a revised training program, Snyder was able to correct a problem she was having with her trailing leg and began recording significantly faster times. The following summer she represented Canada in the 60 metre hurdles at the Tokyo Olympics. Unfortunately, a nasty fall brought a painful end to what could have been a breakthrough performance.

Snyder's fall was not the only disappointment for the Canadians in Tokyo. Twenty-one year old prodigy Bruce Kidd was expected to challenge for at least one medal but failed to advance to the finals in the 5,000 metres and finished in 26th place in the 10,000 metres. At the time, there was talk of injuries, and Kidd was probably not as fit as he would have liked, but years later Kidd gave credence to Percival's pre-Olympic caveat regarding the youth and lack of international experience of the Canadian athletes when he informed Milt Dunnell of the *Toronto Star*, "There is no doubt in my mind now that I had a thorough attack of stage fright – something unparalleled in my experience."

Bill Gairdner's disappointing 11th place finish in the decathlon resulted from a different kind of "attack." Gairdner had not been picked as a medal contender against the powerful Eastern Bloc competitors but was expected to finish in the top eight and earn points for Canada. The evening before his event, Bill and his father went to the Tokyo Hilton to dine thinking that it would be one of the safest places to eat; however, both came down with food poisoning. Back at the Olympic Village, the younger Gairdner became particularly ill and could not find the Canadian team doctor, who was himself somewhere in Tokyo for the evening. When the doctor finally attended to him in the early hours of the morning, he gave Gairdner Laudanum, an opiate, to settle his stomach. Gairdner recovered sufficiently to compete but not well enough to perform at his best. The fact that a Canadian team doctor administered an opiate to a Canadian athlete, only hours before Olympic competition, reveals something about the mixed-up attitude to drugs and sport at that time.

There were numerous Canadian track and field performances to celebrate at the 1964 Olympics. Veterans Bill Crothers and Harry Jerome won silver and bronze respectively, and the younger members of the team generally performed well with Nancy McCredie, Abby Hoffman and Diane Gerace finishing in the top eight in their events and winning points for Canada. This not only represented a dramatic improvement from the results in Rome in 1960, it was Canada's best performance in Olympic track and field since 1932, one that would not be matched in a non-boycott Olympics until 1992 and is still one of the best showings in Canadian Olympic history. Canada won only two other medals in Tokyo. Doug Rogers took silver in Judo and Roger Jackson, who trained with the Don Mills athletes at The Fitness Institute, paired with George Hungerford in the coxless pairs rowing event to win Canada's only gold medal.

In the fall of 1963, Roger Jackson was one of the many young men who aspired to row for Canada in the 1964 Olympics. He had enrolled at the University of British Columbia (UBC) because he saw it as his best opportunity of making the Olympic Rowing Team. But first he had to finish his graduate studies at the University of Toronto. Seeking the best winter training program available, he went to The Fitness Institute where Percival tested him and devised a program specific to the needs of his sport. Jackson worked incredibly hard, and Percival continually modified the program according to his progress. By the time Jackson arrived in Vancouver in April, he was in such good aerobic condition, and his upper body strength had improved so much that he was able to quickly catch up to the other rowers even though they had been on the water since January.

Many factors contributed to the gold medal Jackson and Hungerford won in Tokyo, not the least of which was the coaching legacy of Frank Read and the hard two-a-day workouts the rowers did at UBC, but Jackson calls Percival the "catalyst" to his success. He has stated, "I would not have been part of the Canadian Olympic Team without his (Percival's) encouragement, sound advice and assistance." The individually tailored dry land program devised by Percival was the only one Jackson ever saw as an athlete, and it certainly contributed to his success in Tokyo, but what Jackson remembers most vividly was the atmosphere at The Fitness Institute – working out beside like-minded athletes such as Bill Gairdner, Jenny Meldrum and Nancy McCredie. "The great support and appreciation for hard work helped motivate me," Jackson has stated.

Never before had a diverse group of world class Canadian athletes been together under one roof, working hard at their particular pursuits and feeding off of each other's energy. Percival and MacLennan also fed off this energy and were that much more helpful to athletes as dedicated as Jackson. Jackson remembers one particular winter night when a storm was raging; the streets of Toronto were empty and buses were not running. The isolated Inn on the Park was a desolate spot, but, because it was Jackson's regular training night, he struggled to get there on foot. Jackson walked through the door to find Doug and Lloyd waiting in the lobby and no one else in the building. "We stayed open because we knew you would come," they explained. It was that attitude as much as the scientific equipment and technical expertise that made the opening of The Fitness Institute a turning point in the history of Canadian sport.

Sports Organizations and Individual Athletes

THE FITNESS INSTITUTE WAS HOME to numerous amateur athletes including the St. Catherine's Collegiate schoolboy crew that was preparing to compete in the Royal Henley Regatta in England; top Canadian white-water kayaker, Hermann Kerckoff; Harry Fauquier, a young tennis player Percival had first worked with in 1959 and some of the best flat-water canoeists in Canada. There were also professional athletes and numerous businessmen including Inn on the Park owners, Murray Koffler and Isadore Sharpe. Sharpe was thirty-five years old when he established a daily routine at The Fitness Institute and was soon in better shape than he'd ever been. Sharpe's faith in Percival became so strong that when he broke an ankle while skiing in Europe he refused to let doctors cast the injury because Percival had told him that, for some simple fractures, the hard casts of the day just led to muscle atrophy and most injuries of that type healed better if the body could work to repair itself. Back at The Fitness Institute, Percival personally supervised Sharpe's rehabilitation program and re-taped the ankle every day. Within a few weeks the ankle was almost fully recovered. The extensive use of soft casts and active physical rehabilitation that became common practice some years later offers another example of how Percival was always on the cutting edge of developments in health and fitness.

Amongst the professional athletes who were regulars at The Fitness Institute were Toronto Argonaut football players Dick Shatto and Don Fuell; Frank Mahovlich, Billy Harris and Dick Duff of the Maple Leafs; Gordie Howe and his Detroit teammate, the five foot seven, 145 pound goaltender, Roger Crozier, who was deemed by many to be "too small to long withstand the rigours of NHL play" but who, after a summer at The Fitness Institute, won the Calder Trophy as the 1964-1965 NHL "Rookie of the Year." Percival claimed that there were fifteen NHL players regularly attending The Fitness Institute in 1964. He called them his "secret students" and lamented, "I can't do as much for them as I'd like. If they were to do my exercises during workouts, they would stick out like sore thumbs among their teammates and might get into trouble with their bosses."

Percival's litany of criticisms regarding the NHL had not diminished. When he was called as an expert witness to an inquest into the death of a hockey player whose jugular had been severed by a skate blade, Percival testified, "Hockey is the only major sport in Canada not studying the cause of accidents." He cited his own "Sports College" studies on injuries in hockey and called for "fewer games, more instruction, careful analysis of play, calisthenics for strength, diet, psychology (and) kind encouragement" for developing hockey players. Percival charged that "racehorses are more humanely treated by horsemen than hockey players are by their team management" and repeatedly informed the NHL that it was in its best interest, as well as in the interest of the players, that the NHL adopt a new approach to developing hockey players.

When the Toronto Maple Leafs were in a slump in February 1964, Percival told Paul Rimstead of the *Toronto Telegram* that more hard training was not the answer, that the players were stale and that they required rest and variety in their training if the team was to make a run in the playoffs. The late Carl Brewer referred to this column in his 2006 book, *The Power of Two: Carl Brewer's Battle with Hockey's Power Brokers* (written with Susan Foster). Brewer struggled with depression throughout his career and looked back on his time with the Maple Leafs in the 1960s, wondering how much better it would have been for the more sensitive players, including Mike Walton, Frank Mahovlich and himself, if Punch Imlach had embraced one of Percival's core beliefs that an athlete should be "a happy warrior" because: unless you have the mental outlook that enables you to use your physical abilities to the limit you will never come near your full potential.

Brewer also wished that someone had been paying attention when Percival informed Rimstead that "NHL owners will have to realize some day that hockey players have minds as well as bodies." On numerous occasions, Percival charged that not only did NHL ownership and management see players as mindless; they did everything in their power to ensure that the players would not develop their mental capacities. In April 1961, CBC television broadcast "The Price of Hockey Stardom." Percival debated Stafford Smythe on the subject of education and the Canadian hockey player. He argued that it was morally wrong to treat young teenagers in this manner. Moreover, it was bad for the game of hockey and bad for the NHL because in compromising the natural development of young Canadian hockey players, the NHL was failing to maximize its greatest resource. Neither of these arguments carried any weight with Smythe who defended the tradition of the NHL as best for the players and best for the league. Percival called on the government to enact "legislation that boys cannot be drafted before their high school or university class graduates" – the same system used for decades by the NFL and the NBA – and invited viewers of the program to contact "Sports College" so that he could:

> Organize a campaign to take them (the NHL) out
> of the dark ages and give the game back to the kids
> – give them a chance to get an education and start
> bargaining for their own talent.

Percival became actively involved in creating an alternative for the young Canadian hockey player when he began acting as a scout for Ivy League Universities in the north-eastern United States. These institutions were instrumental in changing the culture of hockey in Canada because the scholarships they granted to Canadian boys helped make American college hockey the first viable alternative to the Canadian junior leagues and allowed Canadian boys, for the first time, to gain a university education while they played hockey.

Inextricably tied to Percival's attempts to free young hockey players from the shackles of the NHL was his continuing effort to introduce modern scientific methods to the training of hockey players in Canada. In 1964, the same year that a delegation of Soviet hockey officials visited The Fitness Institute and shared information with Percival, he published *A Suggested Procedure for Beating The Russians Without Using NHL Personnel*. "The Real Problem… the one we have to solve soon," Percival wrote, was that Canadians still did not believe that "there is something wrong with our present system of developing hockey players in Canada." According to Percival's research, the Russians were "skating an average of four miles an hour faster than NHL players, by actual check, and keeping up the faster pace twice as long or more. . .were better coached in the theory and techniques of the game." It was never Percival's style to sit passively and let the opposition win. He still fervently believed that, if properly trained, Canadian amateurs could defeat the Russians, and he outlined just how it should be done. To those Canadians who argued that it was simply a matter of putting the right professional team out against the Russians, "that we'd only have to throw in the Leafs or Canadiens and chase them off the ice," Percival accurately predicted, "if that's still true – and I have my doubts – it won't be true for more than a year or two."

Drugs and Track and Field

THERE WERE THOSE THAT THOUGHT THE TREMENDOUS SUCCESS of the youngsters who ran for Don Mills came at too high a cost. These critics had yet to give up the idea that Percival's training programs were too demanding and burnt out athletes at a young age. Also, the manner in which the Don Mills athletes came to dominate track meets led to the same jealousy and innuendo that had followed Percival in the 1950s. This time, however, there was also trouble within his own ranks.

For the most part, the Don Mills athletes felt that same sense of commitment and blind loyalty to their coach as the Red Devils had exhibited. This is the same deep emotional bond Kidd and Crothers had with Foot, a bond that was undoubtedly shared by many other East York athletes. When Kidd says that Foot was "like a second father to me" he echoes Bill Gairdner's memory of Percival as a "surrogate father," and Nancy McCredie's description of Percival as "a second dad." This is the faith that all great coaches inspire and Percival, who studied all of the coaching legends, would be the first to point out his lack of singularity in this regard. The obvious downsides to this type of relationship are that should it become stressed and break down, the intensity of emotion must find release. We frequently witness very public examples of this, not just in sports, but in any arena where strong mentor/student relationships evolve.

Amongst the most reverential of Percival's protégés were those that later turned against him: Bob Meldrum, Jenny Wingerson and Nancy McCredie. There was a time when Percival could be found, night after night, on the field after dark holding a flashlight as Meldrum trained. In spite of the extra attention, Meldrum was never quite as successful as some of his Don Mills teammates. When his progress had plateaued, and Percival began devoting more time to other athletes, Meldrum became dissatisfied and looked for someone to blame. Perhaps Percival could have handled it better, but John Hudson, who was close to Meldrum in the early days, believes that Meldrum "could not face up to the fact that he had not been the athlete that he wanted to be – instead of taking a look inside and saying, 'I guess I didn't have it' – he decided it was the coaching." Meldrum said that he quit the Don Mill Track Club. Percival countered that Meldrum was "expelled for conduct detrimental to the club, and that the decision was made by the Don Mills T.C. executive, not by him (Percival) personally."

Jenny Wingerson was one of the best in Canada at shot put, discus and pentathlon, and Percival continued to groom her for international success, but when Nancy McCredie joined the club in 1962, Percival saw the Olympic champion he had always wanted to train. Wingerson found herself receiving less attention and became disillusioned with Percival. She was also engaged to Bob Meldrum, and it didn't take much for him to convince her to join the new Tigerettes Track Club he was setting up.

Nancy McCredie was young, strong and showed great potential. By February 1963, just shy of her eighteenth birthday, Percival was showcasing her talents at the inaugural Telegram Maple Leaf Indoor Games. He even staged a little show of strength for reporters prior to the meet. The newspapers described her as a "shy lithesome lass from Brampton," but Percival knew that "lithesome lasses" were not winning Olympic medals in field events. He began to transform Nancy, and, in the beginning, she co-operated. She says that Percival put her on a 10,000 calorie a day diet with the goal of getting her weight up to 185 pounds. The weight training and practice McCredie had to endure in order to develop strength and technique, as well as mass, was exhausting, but she didn't mind. She later testified, "I thought he was the greatest coach in the world. If he told me to go jump in the lake I'd have done it."

Percival often spoke of the need for "empathy" from a coach. In February 1959, he had written in *Sports College News* that this was "a secret of effective coaching," that the successful coaches "have learned how to place themselves in the position of the other person, to understand just how he is feeling in certain situations." Percival's empathy was one of the trademarks of his coaching that endeared him to the members of the TTFC and the Don Mills Track Club. It is a characteristic that was also appreciated by many other individuals he coached; however, Percival was not one to be contradicted and his huge ego sometimes got in the way of his relationships. By 1964, McCredie had grown a little more mature and independent. She began to chafe at Percival's control over her life. She states that he wouldn't allow her to go to the prom and wanted her to tape the discus to her hand while she wrote exams (McCredie wrote with the hand opposite to the one with which she threw). She also began to realize that she did not enjoy being 185 pounds. Although John Hudson feels that Percival did all that he could under difficult circumstances, Percival probably could have handled things differently at this point. The relationship between athlete and coach became antagonistic, and McCredie became more vulnerable. McCredie grew closer to Meldrum as well as to Bill Crothers. When Crothers and Meldrum convinced her that Percival had tricked her into taking amphetamines, she was deeply hurt. When someone told her that Percival had once moved an infield stake so that her throw registered as a record (an allegation that was groundless and absurd), McCredie "thought she had cheated" and "doubted that her records and victories were real." She said that she quit the Don Mills Track Club soon after the 1964 Olympics, but records show that she represented Don Mills in St. Lambert, Quebec in June 1965, supporting Percival's contention that the club executive expelled her in July 1965 for not following club rules.

By this time, Meldrum, Wingerson and the others in the Tigerette Track Club were sharing the facilities at East York Collegiate with Crothers, Kidd and the rest of Foot's East York club. Meldrum and

Crothers had become, or were becoming, very close – Crothers would act as Bob's best man when Bob and Jenny married in 1966. Crothers does not recall discussing Percival or the use of drugs in the Don Mills Club with Meldrum at this time, nor does he remember sharing any such information with Foot; however, it is clear that the three shared a dislike of Percival, and we know that rumours of Percival and drugs were rife within the East York Track Club.

It was at that track meet in St. Lambert, Quebec, on June 24, 1965, the Eastern Canadian Track and Field Championships where Nancy McCredie was competing as a member of the Don Mills Track Club, that years of innuendo and gossip regarding Percival's athletes and performance enhancing drugs finally bubbled over. Bill Crothers' mother was seated about six rows behind the Don Mills athletes during the afternoon events. That evening she told her son that she had witnessed a Don Mills club official handing out pills that were the same as the pills she had been taking since her recent surgery. Nancy McCredie was one of the competitors that Mrs. Crothers allegedly saw receiving a pill (Nancy also remembers being told that Mrs. Crothers saw her swallowing a pill at the water fountain). The Don Mills Track Club never denied that Mrs. Crothers could have witnessed athletes receiving pills but said that they would have been dextrose (glucose, or fruit sugar) tablets and not the stimulant Dexedrine as Crothers subsequently testified. Soon after the meet, Bill Crothers contacted McCredie and arranged to meet with her at her home in Brampton. He informed McCredie that the pills she had been taking were not dextrose, as Percival had always told her, but Dexedrine.

One of the mysteries of the scandal that began to unfold, which for some reason was not an issue in 1966, was the question of how Mrs. Crothers knew what a Dexedrine tablet looked like. When Bill Crothers was asked this question in 2007, he replied that she would not have known what Dexedrine looked like. The pill she recognized in St. Lambert "would have to have been Tuinal," the sedative that she had been taking. When Crothers was then asked why "…

the Don Mills athletes (were) given a sedative at a track meet in the middle of the afternoon," Crothers responded matter-of-factly, "to take in their hotel room at night after the meet." Admittedly, this interview was held forty years after the fact, and recollections are foggy. But the absurdity of this line of reasoning is consistent with the events that followed.

Since Bob Meldrum was unwilling to discuss details of the affair with the author, we cannot be sure of when or how he became involved, but we know that soon after the meet in St. Lambert there were conversations between Meldrum and Crothers regarding Crothers' belief that Dexedrine and Tuinal were being used on a regular basis by Don Mills athletes. Meldrum began to believe, or began to express, an earlier belief that he, too, had been given amphetamines by Percival. If Percival should be assigned any responsibility for inviting these suspicions it is because he sometimes handed out harmless glucose tablets and told the recipients that the pill would help them run faster, jump higher or throw further. All of the athletes Percival coached knew that he put great faith in the health and the limited performance benefit of taking glucose tablets about twenty minutes prior to intense physical exercise and that they were a regular part of the Don Mills Track Club training routine. So it is hard to imagine that they continued to be an effective psychological ploy. Apparently, however, a few of the Don Mills athletes had come to depend on this psychological boost. No coach would even dream of employing this strategy in the drug-sensitive atmosphere of athletics today, but in the 1960s well-known and respected coaches in a wide range of sports found such subterfuge useful in giving athletes a sense of confidence. The practice naturally engendered suspicion amongst athletes who competed against the Don Mills team – especially the ones who –lost – and led to the rumours and innuendo. It also made the Don Mills athletes susceptible to the suggestion that Percival had been lying when he told them he was giving them glucose.

A plot was hatched to obtain material evidence against Percival. Meldrum, Jenny Wingerson and Nancy McCredie were definitely involved, but Wingerson would testify in court that "Nancy and I were very small parts of this...Mr. Crothers was sort of in charge." It is interesting to note that McCredie remembers becoming closer to Crothers during this period; that he "was like a big brother to me" while Crothers says today, "I never really knew Nancy" and does not remember having anything to do with the plot to acquire a pill as evidence.

The evidence was supposed to come in the form of the heart-shaped Dexedrine tablet Percival was alleged to be supplying to his athletes. The conspirators saw an opportunity in February of 1966. Wingerson and McCredie were chosen to represent Ontario at a dual meet in Vancouver where Percival would be one of the Ontario coaches. Since Meldrum, Wingerson and now McCredie were no longer associated with Percival and Don Mills, they needed someone within the Don Mills club to procure the pill. High jumper Susan Nigh was chosen. While staying at Vancouver's Hotel George, the three young women embarked "on a mission – an adventure" as Wingerson recalls it. They had become convinced that Percival was giving his athletes amphetamines, as Crothers and Meldrum had told them, and therefore believed that they were doing the right thing in exposing him. The girls acquired two pills – or one and one half pills, as it was variously stated – either both obtained by Nigh, or one obtained by Nigh and one by McCredie, again depending on the different versions of the incident. Meldrum and Wingerson said at the time that the pills were immediately given to Crothers, who took them to be analyzed although he does not recall having done so and no test results were ever produced. McCredie stated at the time and later in court that the pills went home in her suitcase and were given to her father, who held onto them until June. She makes the same claim today.

Percival acknowledged that Nigh had advised him that she was not feeling well after the flight to Vancouver, and he had given her a pill upon arrival on Thursday and another on Friday. He said that they were Bonnadette, an over-the-counter air sickness pill that she had taken prior to departure, as well as on other occasions. Furthermore, Percival later argued that he had been aware of the plot: "Therefore, why should I purposely provide evidence?"

If the press knew anything at the time they weren't reporting it. In fact, Bob Meldrum's outburst at the January 18 meeting of the Central Ontario Track and Field Association (COTFA) – of which Fred Foot was the Chairman: "she (Meldrum was speaking of Roberta Picco, one of the Don Mills Runners) will be alright as long as Percival's pep pills hold out" was not found worthy of repeating. Instead, the usual hue and cry was raised by the sportswriters when Percival was passed over as coach of the 1966 British Empire Games team. Even Percival's detractors agreed that, given the success of the Don Mills athletes, this was obviously a snub directed at Percival by Canadian track and field officials. In light of her activities at the time, Nancy McCredie offered a surprisingly passionate defence of her former coach. "He's the best coach in Canada. ... Without him where would I be? ... He would be the best man for the athletes," she told the *Toronto Star*. When the reporter asked if, in spite of their recent differences (quitting the track club), she would like Percival to be her coach at the BEG. "Definitely I would," was her reply.

Percival ignored the snub and immersed himself in his numerous other projects. Clients ranging from the Aurora Highlands Golf Club to the Emmanuel Convalescent Home. The Donwoods Institute (centre for treating addiction) also asked him to draw up physical training programs that would benefit the population they serviced, and the Canadian National Institute for the Blind (CNIB) in Toronto engaged him to conduct classes for their athletic instructors. The CNIB contract led Percival to suggest that "wrestling would be a good activity under supervision" for the visually impaired and inspired a very successful and long-lasting CNIB wrestling program, which included integrated matches with Ontario high school wrestlers, years before there was any other integration of disabled athletes in Ontario. It wasn't wrestling, however, but an unlikely foray into boxing that allowed Percival to shift his focus.

George Chuvalo vs. Muhammad Ali

I N THE BYZANTINE WORLD OF BOXING and its title holders, Ernie Terrell was the reigning World Boxing Association (WBA) champion in the early months of 1966 while almost everyone else recognized Muhammad Ali (Cassius Clay) as the World Champion. The two were scheduled to fight for the undisputed championship on March 29, 1966, at New York's Madison Square Garden. When Terrell's manager, Bernard Glickman, was exposed for connections to organized crime in early February the New York State Athletic Commission cancelled the license, and the fight was shifted to Terrell's hometown of Chicago.

The promoter was Main Bouts Inc. Bob Arum (who would later become one of the most powerful men in boxing) was negotiating the deal, but the President of Main Bouts Inc. was Herbert Mohammad, the son of Ali's manager and Black Muslim leader, Elijah Mohammad. American football great and black civil rights activist, Jim Brown, was also involved in making this the first major boxing match in which black Americans were involved in the deal making as well as in the profits. Main Bouts Inc. was determined that this fight take place on March 29 because Ali was to be called by the draft board on April 1. It is ironic that the man we now consider one of the most erudite and interesting public figures of his era had twice failed to meet the minimum intelligence requirements set by the United States Army. When standards were lowered in November 1965, it became public knowledge that Ali would be reclassified 1A in early April clearing the way for him to be sent to Vietnam.

On February 17th, Ali spoke to the press about his impending meeting with the draft board. He wondered at the motives behind the sudden change in his draft status, discussed openly his association with the Black Muslim movement, insisted on being addressed as Mohammad Ali and questioned America's involvement in the war in Vietnam. When he reportedly said to the press, "I have nothing against the Viet Cong ... the Viet Cong never called me a nigger," Ali became a spokesman and a symbol for disaffected black Americans. To the rest of America and to the Illinois State Athletic Commission, he was a traitor. The license for his bout with Terrell was again withdrawn.

When no American venue could be found Harold Ballard, the owner of Toronto's Maple Leaf Gardens, agreed to host the fight with the stipulation that the winner would fight Canadian Heavyweight Champion George Chuvalo at Maple Leaf Gardens during the summer. Chuvalo's camp was ecstatic. His manager, Irving Ungerman, boasted, "We're ready for Clay (Ali) anytime ... I hope Terrell breaks his arm before March 29, so that we can replace him with George." Terrell didn't break his arm, but someone broke a few of Bernard Glickman's bones and Terrell broke the contract.

On March 12, George Chuvalo signed to fight Mohammad Ali. He had seventeen days to prepare, and no one thought he had a chance. The local press was sceptical; the international press downright hostile. *News of the World* wrote, "It's the night when Muhammad Ali and George Chuvalo, a second class challenger, aided and abetted by the boxing mob, reduce the status of the world heavyweight championship to burlesque. Toronto is a city without sporting shame."

What the press didn't know was that Chuvalo had already begun to train with Lloyd Percival. Records show that Chuvalo's first testing session at The Fitness Institute took place February 22, 1966. Percival devised a training program that would improve the fighter both physically and mentally. Chuvalo had established a reputation as a counter-puncher whose greatest asset was that he couldn't be knocked down, let alone knocked out. Percival planned on turning

Chuvalo into an aggressive, attacking fighter. After the title fight with Ali was announced, Percival intensified the program.

Circuit training was the key to developing the stamina required for Chuvalo's new boxing style, and he loved it. Traditionally, boxers preparing for a fight did road work, hit punching bags and fought sparring partners in the ring. The road work or jogging with some feints and punches thrown in that we have all seen in a myriad of boxing movies could easily have been supplanted by the much tougher and more boxing specific circuit training Percival devised; however, boxing at that time was no less bound in tradition than was hockey. Percival had to contend with Chuvalo's trainer, Ted McWhirter, who wanted no part of Percival's innovations. Another of Percival's innovations was weight training. It seems hard to believe today, but, just as with hockey players from that era, boxers worried that weight training would leave them muscle bound, and boxing trainers considered weight training "ridiculous, if not downright destructive." Percival knew better and employed techniques he had presented in a segment of "Sports College" twenty years earlier to improve the power and the speed of Chuvalo's punches by developing his forearm and triceps.

Percival also introduced to boxing new ideas on nutrition and warming up, but it was in his psychological approach that he hoped to make the biggest difference in Chuvalo. Percival talked to Chuvalo about imaging and stressed words like "aggression" and "tiger" in their sessions together. He told Dick Beddoes that he wanted Chuvalo to be "fierce" and "run over people not around them." Chuvalo says, "I never met anyone like him before and never will again. He was a great teacher. ... It wasn't just the physical thing. ... He dealt with your mind. ... It was the whole package."

We do not know how much three weeks of Percival's program changed Chuvalo as a fighter. We do know that everyone who witnessed the Chuvalo/ Ali fight came away with a newfound respect for Chuvalo's ability as a boxer. The Canadian went fifteen brutal rounds, toe-to-toe with Ali, and proved all of the critics wrong.

Although he lost by a clear and unanimous decision, it was Chuvalo who left most of the sportswriters, from Canada and abroad, tripping over their superlatives and scrambling to apologize for earlier comments. They wrote about Chuvalo's "guts and determination," said that Ali "had never been given a harder, more bruising fight," that Chuvalo had made the champion "dig deep into his capacious bag of pugilistic trickery" and that Chuvalo "proved that he's the toughest man in boxing."

It was the way he came back in the last few rounds of the Ali fight that earned Chuvalo the greatest respect he would ever receive as a boxer. He didn't just stand there and absorb Ali's punishment. Knowing that he would have to score a knockout to win the fight, Chuvalo became the aggressor and brought the Maple Leaf Gardens crowd to its feet. Both boxers were exhausted when they came out of their corners for round fifteen. As the broadcast tapes of the fight dramatically show, it was Chuvalo who "explodes" and "lands four vicious left hands to Ali's jaw before clubbing the champion with a wicked right to the head." For the first time in the fight Ali is seen to be "in trouble." "Chuvalo may have hurt Clay! Chuvalo may have hurt Clay!" screamed fight announcer, Jack Dunphy. The upset was not to be. However, Chuvalo would boast for years that it was Ali who spent the night in hospital while he went out dancing, and the fight has been called "a cultural point of demarcation" for Canada, a moment when "the country stood tall" because of a sporting event comparable only to the 1972 Canada/Russia hockey series, the Gold Medal in hockey at the Olympics in 2002, and the Olympic 100 Metre victories of Ben Johnson in 1988 (at least temporarily) and Donovan Bailey in 2002.

During the 15th round Dunphy also screamed, "Chuvalo is in much better shape than in the fifteenth round of the Terrell fight." Chuvalo still gives credit for his stirring final round to the circuit training devised by Percival, and Ungerman was so impressed with the results that he signed a contract with Percival "to complete the project." Percival said it would require six months but at the end of that time "you won't recognize him (Chuvalo)."

Lloyd Percival vs. COTFA

THE MONTHS OF INNUENDO AND SUBTERFUGE surrounding drugs and the Don Mills Track Club athletes finally surfaced two days after the Chuvalo-Ali fight when Bill Crothers sent a letter to the secretary of the COTFA, which reads:

Dear Don:

I am writing to you because

a) Mr. Pete Beach suggests I must go through my local Track and Field Association.
b) All correspondence is supposed to go through your office.
I regret that I have to do this, but here goes.
I have knowledge, (even proof) that Mr. Lloyd Percival is giving his athletes stimulants (notably dexedrine) and sedatives (for example Tuinal), and that his athletes are accepting them and using these drugs. They have been used for a number of years, including Canadian championships, and international competitions by members of his club, and he was the source of these drugs.
The IAAF and IOC, as well as the affiliated bodies in this country, definitely forbid the use of drugs for the use of increasing athletic performances (to say nothing of the health hazards associated with their use). And I would request, even demands that steps be taken to prevent Canadian athletes from using these drugs.
I would like to add that I am interested not in punitive action, but in preventative action. It would

> bother me to know that adults were resorting to
> the use of these drugs, but it frightens me to know
> that young people (15 or 16 year olds) are being
> given them and are being told that they are like
> glucose.
>   I request that some sort of hearing be held, and
> that some sort of definite action be taken.

The nature of the allegations, especially the association of the two drugs, one an amphetamine and the other a sedative, demonstrates the seriousness of the allegations and the extent to which Crothers apparently believed Percival would use drugs in order to enhance athletic performance. At this time, professional sport, notably football, was under intense scrutiny over the use of amphetamines. In extreme cases, the "high" caused by extensive use of amphetamines had to be counteracted by the introduction of sedatives to bring the athlete "down." The stories in the press during that time about professional athletes and the problems caused by this kind of drug regimen were truly frightening. To associate Percival with these two drugs was sure to cause a sensation.

The COTFA responded to Crothers' letter by summoning him to a meeting on April 4 where he was asked to substantiate his charges. Bob Meldrum was also in attendance. The two men were sufficiently convincing that the committee scheduled a "fact finding meeting" at Toronto's Lord Simcoe Hotel on April 25. According to an official statement released by COTFA prior to the meeting, Percival received a copy of Crothers' letter, was advised that he could bring his lawyer, as well as the Don Mills Track Club doctor and was given the opportunity to request that someone other than Foot chair the proceedings – an opportunity he declined. What is not mentioned in this COTFA statement is that Crothers and Meldrum were required to produce ten notarized copies of statements made by the witnesses they were planning to present. According to Percival, Crothers telephoned him prior to the April 25 meeting to tell him what it was about adding, "If I'm wrong, I'll apologize."

In Crothers' letter, he referred to the IAAF or the International Amateur Athletic Federation that was, and still is, the world body governing amateur athletics, and it was Rule 144 of the IAAF on which this case ultimately hinged. Rule 144 reads:

1. Doping is the employment of drugs with the intention of increasing athletic efficiency by their stimulating action on muscles or nerves, or by paralyzing the sense of fatigue. Their use is strongly deprecated, not only on moral grounds but because of their danger to health.

2. Any competitor who uses drugs as defined above shall be suspended from active participation in amateur athletics for such a period as the council of the I.A.A.F. shall prescribe, and any person aiding and abetting in the use of drugs shall be permanently excluded from any ground where the rules of the I.A.A.F. are in force.

On April 25, Meldrum and Crothers produced four witnesses but no notarized statements. In return for their testimony, the witnesses were promised that they would not be punished for taking the drugs – a clear contradiction of Rule 144 of the IAAF. According to Percival, Crothers "handled the matter 'as the accuser' and presented pills and other evidence" to the committee although Nancy McCredie has consistently denied that they were the pills procured in Vancouver. Since Percival was not accompanied by a lawyer and categorically denied that he was ever given the opportunity, he personally cross-examined his accusers: Bob Meldrum, Jenny Wingerson, Nancy McCredie, Peter Boag and Susan Nigh. Even though their testimony was sufficiently murky and inconsistent to give the directors pause, they decided to move the matter forward.

The Don Mills Track Club immediately drafted a letter appealing the April 25 proceedings and hand delivered it to Foot at his home. When they did not receive an acknowledgement from the COTFA, the Don Mills executive followed up. Foot is reported to have told them that he did not respond because he thought it was a "handbill" not an official document. That didn't stop Foot from showing the letter to George Denniston, Chairman of the Central Branch of the AAU.

On May 2, Don Mills team physician, Dr. William Kerr, who had been unable to attend the previous meeting, was granted an audience by the committee. He brought along Roberta Picco whose ability to train as hard as most men had led to rumours of drug use and prompted Meldrum's outburst in January. Dr. Kerr and Ms. Picco vehemently denied any use of performance enhancing drugs within the Don Mills Track Club. Percival was not allowed to attend this meeting nor would COTFA again grant him the opportunity to face his accusers. At this point, Percival engaged lawyer, George Finlayson, who wrote a letter to Foot objecting to the way the earlier meetings were conducted and to Percival's inability to once more face his accusers.

On May 25, the COTFA tried to unload the problem on the national AAU. By the time the AAU informed the COTFA that they wanted nothing to do with the problem and threw it back in the COTFA's court, the *Toronto Telegram* had broken the story (on May 27, 1966). It was news all across Canada, but nowhere was it as big a story as in Percival's hometown where one front page banner read, "Canada's sports world was rocked today with charges and denials that famed track coach Lloyd Percival has been using drugs in the training of athletes."

Percival's warm relationship with the press initially ensured fair treatment, but there were critics who complained that that relationship, notably with Al Sokol of the *Toronto Telegram*, was "too cozy." They accused Sokol of publishing Crothers' letter only because Percival wanted to make his case before the public rather than respecting the COTFA's desire to deal with it privately. Sokol has stated many times, however, that while it was true that Percival gave him the copy of Crothers' letter that appeared in the *Toronto Telegram* on May 27, this happened only after Sokol had gone to The Fitness Institute to inform Percival that he was going to write a story based on information Meldrum and Crothers had been feeding him for some time and that Meldrum had "aggressively tried to get (him) to write the story and threatened to contact another paper if (he) did not."

The COTFA's first response to the unwanted media attention was to again try to hand the problem over to the AAU. It was rebuffed a second time, and on June 21, they announced the appointment of an impartial, third party to investigate the matter. Percival was encouraged by the direction matters seemed to be taking. From the beginning, he had asked for a proper hearing and had even offered to pay the costs.

Percival continued to work with George Chuvalo after the Ali fight although Chuvalo could see that Percival was troubled, and he saw less and less of him as the track and field scandal unfolded. At the same time, McWhirter was worrying that Chuvalo was becoming muscle-bound and kept telling Ungerman, "you gotta get him (Percival) out of here." On June 24, unbeknownst to him, the registration committee of the Central Branch of the AAU was sitting at a kitchen table somewhere in Toronto deciding his fate while Percival accompanied Chuvalo to New York for his fight against Oscar Bonavena. Bonavena was a big, gangling fighter who, like Chuvalo, was known more for his durability than for his boxing prowess. This was a dull fight, and Chuvalo was slow and sluggish. He claims that he lost because of the New York judges, but the reality was that Chuvalo in no way resembled the boxer who had threatened to hand Ali a 15th round upset and was a mere shadow of the "fierce aggressor" that Percival had watched in sparring sessions leading up to the fight. It is difficult to say whether Percival had not been around enough, whether McWhirter had undermined Percival's program and caused Chuvalo to revert to his former ways, or whether the Bonavena fight was just another of the lurching steps, both forward and backward, that marked Chuvalo's career in the ring. Regardless of the cause, Chuvalo's poor performance brought to an end Percival's foray into professional boxing, and we never found out if six months with Percival would have made Chuvalo a new fighter. Chuvalo was probably more disappointed than Percival. Percival was one of the only people who gave Chuvalo any credit for intelligence and an ability to learn. Chuvalo sensed this and his only regret is that their association was too brief. Percival, however, had other things to worry about. On his return to Toronto, Percival learned that his track club and its athletes had been suspended and his coaching career was in limbo.

After months of waffling, Fred Foot had become decisive and called a June 24 meeting of the registration committee of the Central Branch of the AAU (of which he was also chairman). Present were committee members Mrs. Jesse Lightfoot, Mrs. Doreen Davies, Mr. George Denniston and Mr. Jack Bradfield, none of whom had been present at any of the COTFA meetings. No witnesses were called, and Dr. Terry Kavanagh of the COTFA provided the only evidence: a verbal account of the previous meetings (395 pages of transcript were ignored). At the end of the three hour session, in the presence of invited press but without Percival or any representative of the Don Mills Track Club, George Denniston announced that his committee "was not known for passing the buck" and had found Percival guilty of administering drugs to athletes in the Don Mills Track Club.

In spite of Foot's promise that the witnesses would not be punished, Bob Meldrum, Nancy McCredie, Peter Boag and Susan Nigh were each suspended for two weeks – the fifth witness, Jenny Wingerson never testified to personally using drugs and was not sanctioned. Much tougher sentences had been discussed in the press including the striking of records, the return of medals and longer suspensions. Percival was not a member of the AAU, and therefore could not be suspended. According to IAAF Rule 144, he could have been "permanently excluded from any grounds where the rules of the IAAF were in force." Instead, the Central Branch committee informed the Don Mills Track Club that "it could no longer have an (sic) professional coach," effectively putting Percival out of business without actually naming him in its actions. Because Percival made his living from "Sports College" it was widely assumed that he was paid by the Don Mills Track Club to coach. The fact that he had never been paid one cent for his services really didn't matter in the end.

George Denniston seemed extremely proud of the stand he and his committee had taken and announced, "Our decision may be thrown out in a court of law, right onto the sidewalk, but it will go across the country and stand as far as the AAU is concerned."

Denniston, like Foot, believed that it didn't matter how flimsy the evidence was, Percival was guilty of something and had to be punished. The athletes were back on the track in two weeks, but Percival was left swinging in the wind.

George Finlayson advised Percival that the only way to clear Percival's name and to get everything out into the open was to file a libel suit against the members of the registration committee of the Central Branch of the AAU. On September 23, 1966, Fred Foot, George Denniston, Jessie Lightfoot, Doreen Davies and Jack Bradfield were served with writs seeking $100,000 in damages for libel and slander.

The press had been cautiously on Percival's side regarding the inept and unfair manner in which the meetings and hearings had been conducted. When it came to the charges themselves, however, many were leery of backing the wrong horse. The press and the public were forced to examine the two central figures, Percival and Crothers, and decide whom they believed. On one side was the accuser, Bill Crothers, who had just honoured Canada with a silver medal at the Olympics and was widely respected both inside and outside of the track and field community. In addition, Crothers had recently graduated from the University of Toronto in pharmacology and was, therefore, a creditable witness on the subject of drugs.

Percival, the accused, was certainly well known for being extremely intelligent and knowledgeable, but he was also seen as a bit of a huckster and self-promoter. He had spent years telling anyone who would listen that he knew more than anyone in Canada about the scientific training of athletes and how to help them maximize their performance. It was not much of a stretch for people to believe that he would use performance enhancing drugs to achieve that goal.

Within the track and field community Percival had the reputation of a man who would do anything to win. Those who were jealous of him were likely to assume that he was cheating, and even those who held Percival in high regard wondered how he made these athletes run so fast and jump so high. Bruce Kidd was a member of the East York Track Club but had spent a fair bit of time with Percival because of the great respect he had for Percival's technical knowledge. Kidd had come to believe that Percival had a "win at all costs attitude when it came to technology." Although there were no explicit discussions about performance enhancement, Kidd had distanced himself from Percival because he didn't like the path he thought the coach was following.

Paul Poce recalls that when he and his TOC distance runners watched the petite Roberta Picco train "harder than most of the guys," they concluded "there's something strange here" and that "it was a running gag about Don Mills and pep pills." Poce also informed a reporter that Percival had given him a tranquilizer sometime between 1949 and 1952 – even though the particular drug he referred to was not on the market at that time – but later admitted that he had been caught up in the anti-Percival groundswell and that it wasn't true. Former Red Devil, Murray Cockburn, was an assistant coach with Poce's Toronto Olympic Club at this time. He heard all of the rumours; finding the rush to judgment regarding Percival intolerable, Cockburn resigned his position.

The other athletes in the Don Mills Track Club, as well as the parents and the Board of Directors, didn't believe any of it. They publicly denied any knowledge of Percival giving his athletes drugs.

Murray Cockburn called a meeting at his home in Toronto and invited all of the former members of the Toronto Track and Field Club. Those who attended signed a letter stating that none of them "ever had any idea of using drugs." An attempt was made to have the letter published, but none of the Toronto newspapers would comply. The Don Mills Track Club directors rejected Percival's first letter of resignation; however, facing severe sanctions from the COTFA, they reluctantly accepted the second on July 1, 1966.

Athletes and coaches from outside of track and field who had worked with Percival over the years were shocked to learn that the affair had gone this far. Given Percival's unorthodox methods, his penchant for self-promotion and the envy and jealousy he inspired, the allegations were not entirely unexpected. Still, their knowledge that he had never introduced any illegal substances to them, along with their understanding of his attitude towards competition which did not include cheating, left these men and women unprepared for the judgement. Long-time associates John Hudson, Doug MacLennan and Jim Mossman publicly stated that Percival had only ever advocated natural supplements such as vitamins, oranges and glucose. And Roger Jackson, who would soon be a top sports bureaucrat and one of the most respected men in Canadian amateur sport, submitted an extremely informed and erudite letter to *Toronto Telegram* sports editor, Doug Creighton, praising Percival for his role in preparing Jackson for the 1964 Olympics and weighing in on the drug allegations:

> His (Percival's) positive influence was the direct result of my genuine respect for him as a moral person and responsible citizen. I truthfully state that Mr. Percival never prescribed or suggested that I take stimulants or drugs of any kind under any athletic or non-athletic situation.

At the British Empire Games, held in August 1966 in Jamaica, Canadian track and field athletes won thirteen medals, after winning only seven medals in Wales in 1958 and three in Australia in 1962. The medals were almost equally split between the men and women's teams. Runners and throwers who had been trained by Percival prior to his resignation, but who now trained with John Hudson's Scarborough Track Club, won five of the medals including one of the two gold medals. Former Don Mills athletes also produced seven more top eight placings. No other coach in Canada contributed anywhere near this much to the success of the Canadian team. The winner of the gold medal was shot putter Dave Steen, who also won bronze in discus. When he was interviewed after his gold medal performance, Steen thanked two men whom he said had "influenced him greatly." One was Percival: "I had a coach who took a hell of a beating and I'd like to do him proud, too," Steen announced. When asked if he had consulted with Percival before the Games Steen was careful to reply, "Certainly he talked to me before I left, but as a friend not as a coach."

Percival, his family, his friends and his business associates all suffered due to the bad press. Memberships and other financial opportunities for The Fitness Institute suffered. At the same time, Percival's ability to earn extra income through endorsements and public speaking engagements was severely limited. Sports Illustrated was planning an in-depth study of Percival and The Fitness Institute. A reporter had spent a full week in Toronto following Percival around and interviewing everyone who knew him. When the scandal hit the newspapers, they dropped the story. Percival, Poce and Foot were to be honoured with Government of Ontario "Achievement Awards," but Percival's name was struck from the list a few days before the ceremony.

Those close to Percival talk about the visible toll of the eleven months he spent waiting for his day in court. He worried about his reputation, but he worried even more about his family; he talked about the impact on his daughter, Jan, and on his wife, Dorothy, who "always lived a life of triple tensions, her own, what was happening to me and the effect that had on the way I acted at home." Percival later revealed to the audience of CBC's public affairs radio program "The Day It Is," "This became a very unhappy situation which affected me deeply – emotionally. It affected my family perhaps more so than me because I was at least in a fight. They were on the sidelines." Percival became increasingly isolated by those that weren't sure who to believe and worried that any association with Percival could tarnish their image.

Percival may have been formally barred from track and field in Ontario, but, ever the showman, he still managed to make a big splash in the track and field world. On February 10, 1967, Percival invited reporters and photographers to witness eighteen year old Roberta Picco's attempt to set a new women's world record for distance covered in one hour. The record breaking run took place at the Coliseum building at the Canadian National Exhibition on an unimpeded cement ring behind the seats in the upper promenade, where local track clubs conducted their winter training before there were indoor tracks in Toronto. It was an uncomfortably hard, unbanked surface which Picco had to share with 20 other athletes doing their weekly training. Since this was not an official track and field event it could not result in an official record. Neither could the AAU have any say in the proceedings and no one who participated would be liable for sanctioning. Besides, this was not about setting an official AAU record. This was about showing how good a runner Picco was, how good a coach Percival was and shoving the AAU's nose in it. With the pacing of Jim Irons, one of Canada's top milers, and a last lap push by sprinter Charlie Francis, later to gain fame as Ben Johnson's coach, Picco managed to run nine miles, 1,140 yards and one foot – 1,190 yards more than Irish runner, Ann O'Brien, had run on an outdoor track in Dublin in October 1965.

The trial of Percival vs. Denniston, Foot, Lightfoot, Davies and Bradford commenced on May 17, 1967, before Justice Alexander Stark and a jury of four men and two women. George Finlayson and Percival came very well prepared. Finlayson easily established the damages done to Percival's reputation, as well as his ability to earn a living, and Percival was able to defend himself against the allegations that he administered drugs to his athletes by recalling specific dates and incidents and by producing copies of letters written to the athletes detailing instructions on the use of gravol, glucose and vitamins. Percival also produced literature from "Sports College" that clearly demonstrated his belief in fair play and drug free competition. Moreover, Percival established that scientific data he had been studying since 1944 had convinced him "that the consensus was against their (amphetamines) having any good affect ... that they could only be dangerous."

Percival admitted under oath to administering ten Dexedrine tablets to Nancy McCredie in 1964 when she was recovering from knee surgery and suffering from depression. This action was recommended, and the drug prescribed by Dr. William Kerr, the Don Mills Track Club's physician. Percival testified that this was the only occasion she had been given the drug, and it had no relation to training or to competition. Furthermore, he explained his biggest problem in coaching McCredie was getting her to gain the weight she required if she was to challenge the European and Russian throwers. Anyone with even a limited knowledge of the drug knew that Dexedrine would be counterproductive to this goal. Percival also testified that he gave the sedative Tuinal to Roberta Picco on one occasion – again as per Dr. Kerr's prescription – and that Susan Nigh sometimes received the air sickness pill, Bonnadette, which was available over the counter. These few examples of administering medication all came under doctor's orders. None were in competition. None were intended to enhance athletic performance and in no way, Percival said, did any constitute a violation of Rule 144 of the IAAF. Finlayson and Percival also spent a great deal of time and effort discussing and demonstrating how Percival freely distributed harmless glucose tablets to all of his athletes.

Defence attorney Lloyd Cadsby's cross-examination did nothing to diminish the image of personal and fiscal hardship Finlayson had drawn and failed to cast doubt on Percival's image as an honest and fair coach who abided by the rules. Cadsby's troubles with Percival, however, were nothing compared to the problems he encountered with his own witnesses. Only three witnesses were called: Peter Boag, Jenny (Wingerson) and Nancy McCredie – the two ringleaders, Bill Crothers and Bob Meldrum, "apparently refused to testify." The three young athletes were completely out of their element. They had none of Percival's practice and poise in this kind of hostile environment, seemed poorly prepared, and the evidence they presented was confused and contradictory.

Boag's was the most straightforward testimony presented by the defence. His presence was based on Bob Meldrum's testimony at the April 25 COTFA hearing that: "I asked him (Boag) to look at a number of pills I had on my person ... and (he) immediately pointed at the Dexedrine and said he had been given pills of this type by Percival." At that same April 25 COTFA hearing, Boag was asked if a Dexedrine pill being shown to him was of the type Percival had given to him. He responded, "I cannot say definitely; one resembling it." It should, therefore, have come as no surprise to Cadsby and the defendants when, under cross-examination in court, Boag stated, "I am not in a position to say that the pill I got in 1963 was Dexedrine."

The testimony of Wingerson and McCredie was even more damaging. Wingerson later explained that "They (Boag, McCredie and Wingerson) were not really informed why they were testifying – when the AAU told you to do something you did it." In the courtroom McCredie recalled, "I was so scared on the stand – the lawyer kept asking me questions. I never kept track of these things – I just did what Percival said – I think they made me look like a complete and utter dipstick." Neither of the women was able to substantiate statements made before the COTFA hearings, and they could not even agree that the pills procured in Vancouver were the same ones given to Crothers for testing. Al Sokol had written in May 1966, "It will take a battery of doctors and pharmacologists to determine whether the taking of any of these pills constitutes doping," but neither the pills nor any report of a chemical analysis were produced.

The confusing and conflicting nature of the evidence presented at the different COTFA hearings and meetings in 1965 which should have brought an end to proceedings one year earlier ensured that this trial would end very quickly. After McCredie and Wingerson "admitted they'd made false statements to the AAU hearings into the charges," it was clear to all that Percival would win his suit. Judge Stark consulted independently with the lawyers; the lawyers conferred, and on the morning of May 25, Cadsby read his statement to the court:

> After anxious consideration, the parties to this action have decided that it is in their best interest and in the best interests of amateur athletics in Canada to terminate this lawsuit.
>
> The defendants are now of the opinion that the proceedings that they took, insofar as Lloyd Percival was concerned, were not warranted by the facts.
>
> The defendants are now satisfied that Lloyd Percival did not at any time engage in any doping of athletes ...
>
> Accordingly, the defendants desire to express publicly to Lloyd Percival their apologies for the disciplinary action which they instituted following the meeting of June 23, 1966, and the sending of the telegram on the same day to the Don Mills Track Club.
>
> They propose to recommend the immediate reinstatement of the Don Mills Track Club to affiliation with the AAU of Canada and the acceptance of Lloyd Percival's services as coach, if that is the club's wish.
>
> Lloyd Percival on his part accepts the assurance of the defendants that they at all times acted in good faith.

The defendants were ordered to pay $5,000 to Percival along with the court costs which were later determined to be $12,000. This was nothing like the $100,000 he had been asking for, but Percival had no interest in bankrupting the AAU, and this had never been about money. Some of those close to him wondered why Percival had not let the case continue. There was little doubt that the jury would have ruled in his favour; the settlement would have been higher and the vindication more public. While there were times during the next few years when Percival would wonder the same thing, all he had ever asked for was a fair hearing so he could clear his name, and Percival believed that the trial had accomplished this.

Percival was on the track coaching Don Mills Track Club athletes the same day that Cadsby read his statement. Friends and supporters rushed to congratulate him, and a party was held in his honour that evening. Such was the respect for Percival within the international sports community that amongst the many well-wishers was Nikolai Ozolins, Chairman of the All-Union Committee of Physical Culture and Sport for the Soviet Union, whose congratulatory telephone call from Moscow was taken by Percival during the party.

Nine days later, the Don Mills Track Club made a triumphant return to competition by winning the club title at the Ontario Senior Track and Field Championships, in spite of the defections that had occurred during Percival's absence. That Saturday was Percival's fifty-fourth birthday and "after the final event the Don Mills athletes surrounded their coach and sang happy birthday." It sounds so idyllic – the perfect Hollywood ending, but the reality was very different. Percival later said, "I've never spent a more miserable day. Several athletes (from other clubs) made crude remarks as they passed by me in the infield. And some officials even intimated that they knew the real reason why the registration committee apologized in open court."

The unfortunate reality of our very public legal system is that accusations very often get much more attention than do legal decisions, stay in the public eye for much longer and when the legal argument for the winning side is much more compelling than that presented by the vanquished—we have a tendency to credit the lawyer rather than the evidence. Such was the situation after the Percival settlement. Newspapers, at the time, referred to Percival as having been "vindicated" and "exonerated"; however, over the years the more ambiguous "nothing was proven" has become standard phrase when referring to Percival's libel suit. And he is forever remembered as the man who was "accused of giving drugs to his athletes."

The public was generally content with the ambiguous and those within the track and field community, for the most part, held to the positions from whence they started. It did not help that the COTFA again failed to sanction athletes who admitted in court to having given false testimony before them, even though Foot had touted their integrity stating, "These athletes were all warned of the seriousness of bearing false witness, and if it were proven so, they could be in very serious trouble. They were all aware of this and yet they testified under oath." Bruce Kidd, who has always been a keen observer and a knowledgeable student of Canadian sport, recalls that he "understood that the lawsuit did not settle responsibility," and that a lawyer in the East York club who was involved in the AAU told him and his club mates that "the settlement stops the whole thing but does not absolve Percival." If someone as enquiring and fair-minded as Kidd was willing to accept this interpretation, you can imagine how those who were jealous of Percival and quicker to judge must have reacted.

Percival hadn't anticipated this. He didn't expect everyone to welcome him back with open arms, but he had agreed to the settlement in the belief that people would accept his innocence, and he would be able to return to coaching as before. He was extremely disappointed and frustrated when that did not happen. Percival told John Robertson of *Maclean's* magazine:

> I find it difficult to understand why anyone attaches
> any mystery to what happened in the Ontario
> Supreme Court. I sued them, gave them a chance
> to prove their allegations – the only way they could
> defeat my libel-slander action. And yet, in spite of
> having nearly a year to line it up, their defence fell
> apart and they had to back down. It's that simple.

On October 9, 1967, Percival appeared on the popular CBC television program, "Front Page Challenge." He attempted to establish his innocence and his exoneration but told panellist Gordon Sinclair, "I will probably have to live with the background of the possibility that this really did happen for the rest of my life." Ian Deans, Member of Provincial Parliament for Wentworth, even raised the issue in the Ontario legislature in the spring of 1968 when he accused the Ontario Athletics Commissioner of "failing to do his duty in not protecting the rights of Lloyd Percival." The government did not respond and the matter was dropped. In the fall of 1968, Percival was a guest on "The Day It Is" where he again explained to listeners how he had been cleared of all charges and how the court case caused "personal trauma" and "still affects me very deeply."

Final Retirement from Track and Field

B Y THE TIME OF THE INTERVIEW with "The Day It Is," Percival had retired from track and field coaching, referring to himself as "a perplexed and poorer man." He made the announcement on April 16, 1968, saying that due to his "additional responsibilities in running The Fitness Institute," he was unable to carry on coaching track and field but would continue to act as a consultant to the Don Mills Track Club. Without Percival, however, there could be no Don Mills Track Club and most of the athletes moved over to John Hudson's Scarborough Track Club.

It was true that Percival and Jim Gairdner had begun to plan the building of the new Fitness Institute in Willowdale, and Percival was extremely busy, but there was no other point in his life when Percival let circumstance or other people dictate his decisions. It is abundantly clear that he was very tired, and the accusations of athletes he had nurtured, the lawsuit and his failure to completely clear his name had left Percival with no appetite for coaching a track and field club. In addition, Percival's mother had died on March 14, only one month before he announced his decision to retire. It seemed that, for the only time in his life, the fight had been knocked right out of Lloyd Percival.

Percival's contribution to track and field while coaching the Don Mills Club cannot compare with what he did for track and field in the TTFC era. He had started with nothing in 1946; no one else had contributed anything comparable to that which he brought to the sport during those years, and there is no question that without him, the sport would not have matured in Canada as dramatically as it did. By 1960, track and field in Ontario was on solid footings, and there were other excellent coaches and officials who raised the standards of track and field throughout Canada and helped make Canadians a force in international competition for the first time since 1932. In spite of this, Percival still coached the strongest track club in the country and sent more athletes to international competitions than any other Canadian coach. Along with Vancouver sprinter Harry Jerome, a few of Fred Foot's middle distance stars and some of Paul Poce's long-distance runners, it was Percival and his athletes who raised Canada's international stature in track and field, and for a few glorious years made track and field a major spectator sport at home. He was still the greatest technical innovator in Canadian track and field and his absolute refusal to accept mediocrity helped drive his athletes and those who competed against them to heights they would not otherwise have attained.

The national and international success enjoyed by the individuals within the Don Mills Track Club was as important to the future of these young men and women as the experiences of TTFC members had been in the 1950s, and, although his personal influence may not have been as pervasive in the 1960s, many of these athletes also credit Percival for having a profound effect on their lives after their competitive careers were over. Bill Gairdner and Bill Heikkila are amongst those who still employ coaching methods learned from Percival and believe that this gives them an advantage over other coaches. Heikkila calls Percival "one of the two great mentors" in his life, and Gairdner says that "I hear Lloyd talking to me every day." Roberta Picco (Angeloni) wrote that Percival "taught me many things about myself and people ... encouraged me to compete and to strive ... (and) taught me not to fear failure, or success." Even Percival's accusers remember the life lessons that he imparted to them. Jenny Wingerson acknowledges that "He was a great coach. He taught me that 99% of the battle is mental. I have used that ever since," while Bob Meldrum tries to remember the good times more than the bad and says that, "I owe a lot of what I learned in life from him."

Percival's influence beyond the confines of his track club included cases where he directly impacted upon the success of some of Canada's greatest track and field athletes.

Abby Hoffman was coached by Paul Poce, and Percival's own protégé, Roberta Picco, was emerging as Hoffman's main rival on the track, but that didn't deter Percival when he saw that Hoffman needed help. According to one source, Percival witnessed Hoffman struggling in competition and suggested to Poce that she might be suffering from an iron deficiency. Blood tests showed that Hoffman was indeed anaemic, and iron supplements were prescribed.

In the case of Canada's first sub-four minute miler, Dave Bailey, Percival intervened twice. Four months prior to running his 3:59.1 mile in San Diego on June 6, 1966, Bailey talked to Percival about vitamins. Percival referred Bailey to Dr. Kerr, who did some blood tests and corrected what was an ineffective, and possibly harmful, vitamin regimen that had been devised for him. But Percival's most important contribution to Bailey's success resulted from a more subtle intervention a few years earlier. In 1964, Percival and Bailey were part of an Eastern Canadian team that was traveling by train to a meet in Vancouver. At one point, the two were seated side by side. It was very unusual at that time for a coach, even Percival, to give advice to an athlete from another club. On this occasion, however, Percival turned to Bailey and imparted a few simple words:

> You know what your problem is Dave? You worry too much about where you are going to finish. Just concentrate on your execution.

How often during the 2010 Winter Olympics in Vancouver did we hear athletes and coaches talk about focusing on the process, not on the results? It has become a mantra for the modern day athlete. Fifty years ago, Percival was speaking a different language, but Bailey got the message. He says today:

It crystallized everything for me and changed my
whole approach to competition. I learned that
you cannot control the result – only the process.
… This made me more effective – made me a lot
better racer as a result. I used this ever after in my
racing and in my coaching.

Bruce Kidd had a tremendous amount of respect for his coach,
Fred Foot, and his understanding of strategy and tactics but recognized that Foot's knowledge of physiology was limited. He saw
something different in Percival – something akin to his own deep
curiosity – and spent a lot of time with Percival discussing the physiological aspects of running. Kidd found that he really appreciated
Percival's "scientific, systematic approach." Kidd feels that he was
"privileged" and "lucky" to have these moments and says, "I would
be the first to say that I learned a tremendous amount."

Members of the TTFC who attended American universities
on athletic scholarships introduced Percival's coaching methods to
American athletes to a degree we will never be able to measure. To
a much lesser extent, this also took place in the 1960s. We do know,
however, that Willie Davenport, one of the greatest athletes in the
history of United States track and field, visited Percival in Toronto
in 1964. At the time, he was a good young hurdler; a few months
after meeting with Percival, he was American champion and on his
way to becoming a legend.

Larry Dunn was an American who came to Canada and trained
with the East York Track Club in the early 1960s. While there,
he became friends with Jim and Marian Snyder. It wasn't long
before the draft board called him back home, but he returned to
Canada on a regular basis and usually stayed with the Snyders.
In 1964, after the Snyders had left East York Track Club to train
with Percival, Dunn brought his friend, Willie Davenport, one of
many fine young American hurdlers hoping to gain a spot on the
United States Olympic team that summer. Davenport was watching
Marian Snyder race one day and became intrigued by her technique

with her trailing leg – the technique Percival had recently taught her. Davenport was invited to a Don Mills training session where Percival taught him the same technique and introduced him to the workouts he had designed to help Snyder incorporate it into her hurdling. Willie Davenport became "the surprise winner" of the 110 metre hurdles at the U.S. trials that summer and was the favourite to win the gold medal in Tokyo. A thigh injury kept Davenport out of the medals in 1964, but he won a gold medal in 1968 as well as bronze in 1976, was recognized as the best American hurdler of his era and participated in his fifth Olympics when he was named to the American four-man bobsled team in 1980.

While it was true that the controversy surrounding Percival had left a cloud over The Fitness Institute, limiting business opportunities, curtailing speaking engagements and dissuading some athletes from being associated with him, Percival never stopped working with many of Canada's best athletes.

Peter Burwash

Isadore Sharpe's newfound enthusiasm for sport included tennis lessons from one of Canada's best young professionals, Peter Burwash. Sharpe was immediately impressed with the young man's enthusiasm and positive attitude. After learning of Burwash's desire to try the international professional circuit and the financial investment that was required, Sharpe offered to buy Burwash the worldwide airplane ticket that would enable him to play the tour for one year. There were no strings attached. Sharpe just wanted to be kept abreast of how the young tennis player was doing. Sharpe says that this was an easy offer to make because he "always felt that Peter would contribute to society."

Sharpe introduced Burwash to Lloyd Percival, and the chemistry was immediate. While Percival was usually generous with his time, there is no question that he favoured some athletes. It was not always the most talented athletes, but it was always the athletes who showed a keen interest, not just in training, but also in gaining an understanding of their bodies and of their minds. Percival delighted in telling people that most potential Olympic champions were out walking the streets, oblivious to their potential. As he stated in one of his last interviews, "The best athletes do not come from 'the top echelon of physical talents,' but from 'achiever personalities.' " Peter Burwash exemplifies the achiever personality.

While Burwash's competitive spirit was fired in the hotbed of Canadian hockey (he was drafted by the St. Louis Blues, but an injury forced him to give up hockey) he won his first tennis tournament at age twelve on "heart, guts and speed." These would become Burwash's trademarks during his professional career. It fell to Percival to supply the missing ingredient – incredible fitness.

Percival first developed fitness routines specific to tennis when Harry Fauquier came to him a couple of years earlier. Fauquier spent one hundred of the last one hundred twenty days at The Fitness Institute before he joined the professional tour but worked out on his own for the remainder of his career. Peter Burwash, on the other hand, became one of the most recognizable faces in Percival's gym for many years.

Percival frequently supervised or monitored Burwash's fitness routines. "He was tough but never mean. I liked it," Burwash says today. Percival also supplied him with an exercise regimen to follow while he was on tour. The key ingredient, missing in any other fitness program for tennis players, was the tennis specific exercises Percival prepared for Burwash. During his seven year professional career, Burwash claims to have been the fittest man on tour: "I never tired in a match. I always stayed fresh until the end." Percival had Burwash do "an enormous amount of work on wrist and leg strength as well as cardiovascular," and he broke down the movements and physical requirements of the game before creating routines to improve Burwash's backhand, forehand and serve. Percival also insisted that Burwash do all of his routine from the left side as well as from the right, in order to develop balance and so that "if necessary,

Gary Mossman

he could play left-handed." Burwash enjoyed an injury free career – almost unheard of among tennis professionals – save for tennis elbow related to serve mechanics that pre-dated his training with Percival. Even then, Percival's program came through. Burwash was able to practice left-handed while recovering from surgery and appreciably speed up the rehabilitation process. Burwash recalls that Percival "thought of everything" and, just as importantly, "he always explained why I was doing things."

Nutrition was one area where Burwash did not need any help. He has always been health conscious and, since 1969, has been a strict vegetarian. In 1970, Burwash arrived at The Fitness Institute for his annual battery of tests. A tough tournament schedule and airline problems had left him suffering from fatigue and jet lag. He feared that he would not score well. When Percival read the results, he surprised Burwash by asking, "What have you been doing? These tests are fantastic." Burwash informed Percival of his new diet. Percival had strong ideas on nutrition, and they did not include vegetarianism. But he kept an open mind and, in light of the test results, supported Burwash in his choices. This was very important to their relationship, as Burwash's dietary decisions became a central component of the lifestyle he continues to this day.

By the 1970s, Peter Burwash was one of the fittest athletes Percival had ever tested. Percival told him that he "had the best stress test score of anyone at The Fitness Institute." When the Canadian Davis Cup Team was tested in 1970, Burwash registered a VO2 (maximum oxygen) uptake of 72 ml/kg/minute, a high score for any athlete. Of the other Davis Cup Team members, Mike Belkin had the next highest at 49. The training Percival devised, combined with the effort Burwash was willing to put into his program and the "never say die" approach that had impressed Isadore Sharpe, brought Burwash seven productive years on the professional tennis circuit and that 1970 Davis Cup Team – the only one that Percival was asked to work with – produced one of Canada's most significant international tennis victories.

222

After retiring from the professional tour in 1974, Burwash founded Peter Burwash International (PBI) which now manages tennis operations at more than sixty clubs and resorts around the world. The tremendous success of PBI is built on quality teaching and an instruction program that demands a high degree of consistent professionalism. It also succeeds because of an appreciation of individual needs and a refusal to accept mediocrity – principles that were strongly reinforced because of Burwash's work with Percival. To this day, Burwash carries around a red pen to make notes on anything that strikes him as important, just as he witnessed Percival do whenever they were together. Lloyd Percival would be very proud that his former student has been recognized as "one of the world's best tennis coaches," as "the smartest man in tennis today" and was acclaimed by *Tennis Industry Magazine* as "one who has changed the game." He is the author of ten books and is an internationally sought after motivational speaker. His 1995 Education Merit Award from the International Tennis Hall of Fame paid homage to the work he has done bringing free tennis instruction to "prison inmates; abused children, people in wheelchairs, deaf and blind players and children with varying physical challenges." Percival helped him gain an appreciation of sport as a means to an end, not as an end in itself. Burwash himself has taken that ideal, stretched it much further into the realm of social responsibility and has made a significant contribution to society, just as Isadore Sharp predicted. Burwash says today that there are "three pillars of any success" he has had in life. His family is the first. Then, "side by side, stand Issy Sharpe and Lloyd Percival."

George Knudson and Al Balding

Prior to Mike Weir's victory in the 2003 Masters Tournament, George Knudson and Al Balding were the biggest names in the history of Canadian men's professional golf. Knudson spent eleven years on the tour and was named "Golfer of the Twentieth Century" by the Canadian Professional Golf Association (CPGA). He just missed usurping Weir as the first Canadian male to win a "Major" when he finished second in the Masters in 1969. Not until his tenth year on the PGA Tour, at Scottsdale in 2007, did Weir equal Knudson's career record of eight official Tour victories; he has been pursuing the elusive number nine ever since. Weir's highest finish on the annual list of top PGA Tour money winners came in his break-through 2003 season. The previous best ranking by a Canadian was Balding's sixth-place finish in 1957 – two years after he became the first Canadian to win a PGA Tour event. Knudson and Balding had one thing going for them that Weir lacked – Lloyd Percival.

Knudson and Balding were already successful golf professionals, in Canada and in the United States, prior to joining The Fitness Institute, but Percival had a major impact upon their golf careers. Knudson had been a professional since 1958 and a PGA Tour regular since 1961. With four tour victories already to his credit, he regularly contended for tournament titles. From tee to green, Knudson was one of the very best – he was ranked number two on the tour in 1966. On the green, however, every putt was an adventure – that same year he was ranked number 120 in putting. Jack Nicklaus reportedly said that Knudson had "a million-dollar golf swing and a 10 cent putting stroke."

Knudson turned to Percival in October 1966 partly because of his putting woes, but mostly to address problems with fatigue. He said, "I couldn't play more than a couple of weeks in a row without becoming physically and emotionally depleted. ... At 135 pounds, I had neither the durability nor the strength to play the way I was capable of." The program Percival put together for Knudson was designed to "control tension, eliminate fatigue and maximize strength." It targeted flexibility and strength and included aerobic exercises as well as weight training for Knudson's upper and lower body so that he would develop "the power he needed and the stamina needed in the final round of a demanding course."

By the spring of 1968, Knudson carried one hundred and seventy pounds on his five foot ten inch frame. He was still lean but was much stronger, and it showed. Arnold Palmer remarked after a Knudson tee shot, "Either you're getting stronger, or I'm getting older." Knudson said, "I've never hit the ball so well and I've never been in better shape. ... I never knew there were such things as specialized golf exercises until I went to Lloyd Percival last winter. I feel so great it isn't real." Knudson was in contention for seven straight weeks, earning three top ten finishes in the first five events. The big payoff came in Arizona where Knudson became the first non-American to win back-to-back tour events. In Phoenix, Knudson was brilliant from tee to green and held on to a one-shot lead through the final round, in spite of requiring 65 putts through Saturday and Sunday. Knudson credited his new found endurance to the training he was doing at The Fitness Institute with Lloyd Percival.

At the second Arizona tour stop in Tucson, Knudson's strength and stamina were again equal to the task. Mentally, Tucson was even more demanding than Phoenix had been. After the third round on Saturday, Knudson said, "I felt myself tightening up so much that I creaked when I moved." Knudson talked to Percival on the telephone, as he did almost every day that spring, before shooting 65 to overcome a four stroke deficit. But it required all of the physical and psychological resources that Percival had helped Knudson develop. Knudson recounted his walk to the 18th tee:

> I was thinking on the way over that a four would win or at least tie, but the hole has water on each side of a fairway that slopes both ways. I was shrugging my shoulders to get that relaxed feeling but thought that I needed something else. So I did the monkey slump and that really cooled me. I was ready.

The shoulder shrug and the monkey slump were relaxation techniques that Percival had taught Balding and Knudson. The former involves shrugging your shoulders up as high as possible, holding for several seconds and then relaxing. As the shoulders drop, the head comes forward to relax the neck muscles. Percival instructed Knudson and Balding to do this "ten times, several times a day and before and after every shot." As for the monkey slump, Percival describes it in *RELAXATION is easy*:

> Stand upright, feet comfortably apart, arms
> hanging loosely at your sides. Then let your head
> fall forward as far as possible. Then, gradually start
> to drop your head and upper body toward the floor,
> arms hanging loosely like an ape. Each time you
> slump down a little more, let your knees bend a bit.
> Continue your slump until your upper body is bent
> right over and your hands are touching the floor.
> Do 4 or 5 times. Really dangle!

Doing the shoulder shrug during a round of golf would not have raised many eyebrows, but doing the monkey slump in front of the other golfers and thousands of spectators speaks to the faith he had come to place in Percival's teachings. "Maybe those watching thought the sun had got to me," he said, "but I knew I had to get loose."

Knudson recorded a four on the 18th hole and won his second tournament in as many weeks but left Tucson physically and emotionally exhausted. He may have learned how to handle the weekly grind of the tour, but he hadn't learned how to deal with the pressure that comes with winning. At the Canadian Open held at Toronto's St. George's Golf and Country Club in July, Knudson was the centre of attention, and the pressure was on for him to win his home Open. The scrutiny intensified when he evaded the press and the other golfers on the practice range and drove to The Fitness Institute after a disappointing opening round 75 – a round he said "would have destroyed the old George Knudson." Knudson rallied to shoot a 69 and a 64 before his putter once again betrayed him, and he finished seven strokes behind winner, Bob Charles.

Like Knudson, Al Balding had felt the pressure of becoming the first Canadian to win the Canadian Open since 1954 when he was in contention in the 1961 Open, also held at St. George's. And, more recently at Toronto's Glen Abbey in 2004, Mike Weir learned that even a victory in the Masters cannot fully prepare a Canadian golfer for the psychological challenge of winning his national Open. Knudson has said of his experience, "Maybe I tried too hard. But being able to live it and accept it – that was the most important thing." His performance showed just how far Percival's program had taken Knudson.

The final feather in Knudson's cap for the 1968 season came in Japan where he and Balding shared a victory in the Canada Cup (now the World Cup), an international, two-man team competition; however, in this one, George was just along for the ride. He shot a pedestrian 295 over four days while Balding was brilliant, shooting 274 and capturing individual honours.

Al Balding became a regular at the Institute after Knudson introduced him to Percival sometime in the fall of 1966. In that pivotal 1968 season, Knudson insisted that Balding accompany him to each session. They would head off at five-thirty in the morning, do their workouts and have a massage. Percival was usually around to check on their progress and often sat down with them for a chat. Although the two golfers spent a lot of time together during these years and got along well, they had contrasting personalities and were never close. Percival recognized this and related to each differently. For the high-strung Knudson, he was much more than a strength and fitness trainer; he was a confidante and an ally in the golfer's life-long battle with personal demons. Knudson spent long hours on the telephone with Percival, and it was not uncommon for Percival to be awakened at three o'clock in the morning by a call from Knudson. The nature of the relationship was reflected in the training programs

Percival developed for Knudson and were like none of the hundreds of programs he produced for other athletes.

It was common practice for Percival to provide a special training program for an athlete in competition. It was not common, however, for him to include clear and detailed instructions on how the athlete was to organize his or her day. For Knudson, these details included physical exercises and visualization drills to do before and after he got out of bed, others for tournament and practice and a still different routine for the evening. Percival's visualization techniques are commonplace in all sport today, but Percival was the first to introduce a detailed, structured visualization practice to golf. He instructed Knudson:

> In your mental practice (and do it every day) pick
> out every shot you are likely to ever make and
> make it in your mind – see it, feel it. If possible
> draw a picture ... then close your eyes, go through
> the action and make it. Remember – the more
> often you make all shots (physically and mentally)
> the more likely you are to make them.

There was a constant push from Percival to build up Knudson's confidence through routine and through positive reinforcement. Percival told Knudson that he wanted him to "feel 'right' more often," and he even wrote him using the third person: "This Is The Time To Get Control, The Image of Yourself, That Will Allow Knudson To Play Like Knudson – And That Is All You Need To Make A Little History. You Know It, I Know It – Let's Do It." Almost all golfers today work with a psychologist, and some have their "mental coach" with them at tour events. Tiger Woods' psychologist frequently caddied for him when he was dominating junior tournaments. But the phenomenon is a recent one. Although Percival never accompanied either Knudson or Balding at a golf tournament, it is almost certain that theirs was the first such relationship in the history of professional golf.

With the more laid-back Balding who served his country in WWII and had worked as a truck driver before joining the PGA Tour in 1955 when he was thirty-one years old, Percival became a buddy. Balding won the 1955 Mayfair Open that first year and followed it up with two more victories in 1957. Balding also won five CPGA championships although physical problems plagued him throughout his career. In 1965, he had the first of three surgeries to repair shoulders that had first been injured during WWII. In 1966, Percival introduced exercises to strengthen Balding's shoulders and improve his all-round fitness.

Balding's performance in the 1968 Canada Cup was all the more remarkable because he was forty-four years old, a very advanced age for a golfer on the PGA Tour even today. The Seniors Tour did not exist as yet, and older golfers generally retired or faded away. He remains the oldest golfer ever to have won individual honours in the World Cup, and the physical fitness routines he learned from Percival served him well over the years. In spite of his various ailments, Balding enjoyed some success on the Seniors Tour when it did come along. In 2000, at the age of seventy-six, he won the Canadian Seniors Title shooting a remarkable 70 / 70 / 70, six strokes under par and six strokes less than his age in each round. And at a PGA Seniors Tour event two years later, Balding shot a 66, twelve shots less than his age, a feat unmatched in tournament golf.

Sports psychologist, Dr. Richard Keefe, in his book *On the Sweet Spot: Stalking the Effortless Present* (2003), describes the relationship between a golfer and his psychologist:

> One of the unspoken yet essential components
> of a successful sport psychology consultation is
> that, as the golfer continues to open up about his
> experiences on the golf course, he'll begin to refer
> to the psychologist in his mind while he is playing
> and be comforted by this image of someone who
> wants him to succeed, grow and develop.

Balding related an incident at the 1968 World Cup in Japan which clearly demonstrates that Percival had taken on the role of psychologist for Balding as well as for Knudson. Before he headed to Japan, Percival worked with Balding on techniques for staying calm and relaxed during the tournament and informed Balding most emphatically, "I'll be there with you." With only ten holes to play on Sunday, Balding was feeling the pressure. He recalls quite vividly that while walking up a hill on the ninth fairway he "looked up and saw Percival's face in the crowd. It was just a flash." The image of his coach back in Canada helped Balding realize that he was playing too quickly and was in danger of losing control of his emotions. He remembered that Percival had taught him that it was not just a bad shot that could lead to tension. Too much positive energy could leave you "over-activated" and playing too fast. Dr. Keefe also discusses this condition:

> When attention is excited, it is almost impossible
> to keep the mind focused on a single object; your
> thoughts wander and jump through a forest of
> ideas, feelings, hopes, and anxieties.

Balding was able to refocus. He did some shoulder shrugs, slowed himself down and shot a 33 on the back nine to close out victory for himself and for the Canadian team.

Percival's training methods were not a magic cure, but his scientific and psychological approach to a sporting activity previously ruled by imitation and tradition made Knudson and Balding better golfers and helped them compete with the best in the world. Knudson once said to a reporter, "I can't help wondering what might have happened if Percival had got me at 18 instead of 30." This wisdom is even more applicable to Al Balding, who was introduced to Percival when he was forty-two. While Knudson began spending less time with Percival after he realized that the success he had dreamt of didn't bring him inner peace, and he turned more and more to teaching, Balding continued to be a regular at the gym as well as in Percival's office. They were together the day before Percival died discussing a golf instruction book they were to produce together.

It would be decades before Percival's innovations were widely adopted by professional golfers. Today, however, every professional golfer has at least one golf coach and one physical trainer; work on the practice range doesn't begin until the gym workout has been completed, and it is followed by a treatment from the massage therapist. Afterward, there is a session with the sports psychologist. It sounds a lot like a typical morning at The Fitness Institute in 1968.

Skiing

Eddie Creed's fifteen year old son, Jack, was the first competitive skier to work with Percival soon after The Fitness Institute opened, but it was not until two of Jack's female teammates from the Ontario Ski Team showed up in 1967 that Percival began to impact upon the sport.

Diana Gibson came first, seeking treatment for an injury. She was joined by Judy Crawford, her friend and classmate at Branksome Hall, the private girls' school Percival had attended when he was a small boy. The two grade nine students became regulars at The Fitness Institute, and Percival introduced them to personalized strength training when it was almost unheard of for skiers, even for the European men. Crawford remembers Percival being "very knowledgeable, but never overbearing. ... (he) would talk to you at your own level, without talking down to you." This facet of Percival the coach was sometimes overlooked during this stage in his career. His ability to inspire young people at the same time as he empowered them had been a key to the success of his Red Devils Track Club, and it continued to be a key to his success in the 1960s and 1970s.

Gibson and Crawford went to the national training camp at the Kokanee Glacier in British Columbia in 1968. But for an injury to

Gibson, both would have made the National Ski Team that year, and they credit Percival with supplying the physical conditioning that put them over the top. For Roger Jackson, Percival had helped to provide the strength and endurance to overcome the advantage West Coast rowers gained through a longer season on the water; for the skiers, Percival's dry land training helped compensate for the western skiers' extra time on the hills. In both cases, the athletes were fully prepared because of Percival's innovative and scientific approach to athletic training.

Hockey

NHL goalie Dave Dryden showed up at The Fitness Institute in 1967 to work on his conditioning and became one of Percival's prize pupils. Not blessed with as much natural talent as his famous younger brother, Ken, Dave Dryden enjoyed an eighteen year NHL/WHA career based on hard work. As well as the usual fitness program, Percival devised a board with a collection of coloured lights that was hung on the wall in front of Dryden. The lights flashed in random sequence, and Dryden was required to hit each light with one of his hands as soon as he saw it. His reaction time (both with and without goalie gloves) was measured and recorded. The device was used to both test and to improve the goalie's ability to react. In the 1990s, a commercial version of Percival's machine, developed without any input from or even knowledge of Percival's work, hit the market and found its way into NHL training rooms.

Other NHL players who started showing up at The Fitness Institute usually came for short-term treatment of a particular injury but still had to keep their attendance a secret. Carl Brewer was an exception. He had already established himself as a rebel whose talents overshadowed his idiosyncrasies, and he had no trouble publicizing Percival's assistance with his return to the NHL in 1968. And there was one general manager who had the courage to challenge the collective wisdom of the NHL.

Wren Blair had gone from the Whitby Dunlops to the Boston Bruins organization before being named general manager of the Minnesota North Stars, one of six new teams set to join the NHL in 1967. Blair concluded that by concentrating on conditioning, his roster of aging veterans and untried rookies could become competitive. He hired Lloyd Percival not because of what Percival had done for him in 1958, but because Blair recognized that the Russians were far ahead of Canadians in terms of physical conditioning, and Percival was the leading expert on Russian hockey training.

Percival's three phase program – off-season, pre-season and regular season – emphasized tension release and strength with "particular attention … paid to the groin and shoulder areas where injuries are common and cost a player numerous lost ice hours." Rest and variety were also stressed, and Percival sought to recognize the individual needs of each player because he said while "the science of conditioning is knowing all the mechanical means of creating conditioning, the art is knowing how to schedule it and knowing the psychology of each person so the individual gets precisely what he needs." As always, the importance of a proper diet was emphasized. Although Percival recognized the uphill battle he had been fighting against the tradition of the pre-game steak and suggested that "if a player has a psychological quirk about a game day steak, we don't try to talk him out of it, but we advise him to remove all of the fat. Furthermore we advise that the meat be minced since it is easier to digest."

The North Stars finished the 1967-1968 season just four points out of first place in the West Division and lost in overtime, the game that sent the West Division representative to play for the Stanley Cup. During that season, the North Stars lost only twenty-three player games due to injury, considerably less than any other team in the league that season or any other season in the history of the NHL. Percival's dedication to injury prevention was the major reason and was a significant factor in the decision to bring him back for the 1968-1969 season. Unfortunately, the North Stars were not as successful in their second season. When the team began to lose, players and management looked for reasons and anything that was a little different was suspect. Blair remembers thinking that the players weren't paying attention to Percival anymore: "When they started to get sick of it, I let it go." By the end of the season, Percival was gone and the North Stars were out of the playoffs.

As a coach and as a general manager, Wren Blair was never afraid to go against the grain and try something the rest of the hockey people rejected. Unfortunately, this did not include a long-term commitment to Percival's program. The thing that Blair, along with Jack Adams in the 1950s and any other coach who introduced some aspect of Percival's teachings to the NHL, failed to understand was that Percival's program was not a gimmick like pyramids under the bench or wearing a lucky hat. It was a system that had to be learned by management and players, had to be introduced into every aspect of the training and development of the hockey players and allowed to evolve over time. These men lacked the insight and foresight required to employ Percival's teachings as an integrated and holistic program.

Canada's First Cardiac Rehabilitation Program

PERHAPS THE MOST IMPORTANT CONTRIBUTION made to the health and fitness of Canadians by Percival and his staff at the original Fitness Institute was the rehabilitation program initiated with a group of cardiac patients. Doug MacLennan can't recall an exact date when cardiac rehabilitation became one of the services offered. It was not in the original plans, but MacLennan and Percival always sought to accommodate the needs of the membership. The middle aged businessmen who joined The Fitness Institute had a number of health concerns, often related to lifestyle, and they included heart problems. MacLennan recalls Percival consulting with Dr. Kerr regarding some of these members before former Green Gael lacrosse player, Dr. Charles Bull, just embarking on his career in sports medicine, began consulting the eight to ten men who required cardiac rehabilitation at any one time. Evidence can be found in a script for a "Sports College" television pilot from 1963 featuring Canadian Heart Foundation director, Murray Robertson, taking part in a "scientifically designed program to test the value of exercise in re-conditioning his heart, in improving its functional fitness, to see if exercise can be of value in preventing heart disease." There is also a photograph of Robertson hooked up to a heartometer at The Fitness Institute in the April 18, 1964, edition of *Maclean's*.

According to an interview Jim Gairdner gave in 1984, Percival's first cardiac rehabilitation patient was the elder Gairdner himself: "This was one of our earliest concepts. It started when I had a 'cardiac alarm' and we discovered that there was no place to go in Canada I could be tested and put on a program." Jim Gairdner was of the generation that survived the trauma of WWII and prospered in the economic boom that followed. The hard living that went hand in hand with the hard work that made them successful caught up to so many of these men. They became Canada's "captains of industry" before they became charter members of The Fitness Institute, and Jim Gairdner was one of the earliest casualties of an unsustainable lifestyle. With Percival's help, he initiated dramatic changes and enjoyed an extremely active and healthy life until his death in 1996 at the age of 77.

In anticipation of a move to larger premises in 1968, Percival issued a long press release extolling the successes of The Fitness Institute including the "cardiac recovery program" and giving a detailed description of well-established protocols, safety precautions and technical aids used for each member's individually designed rehabilitation program. These included prior screening and approval by the member's cardiologist, continuous monitoring and evaluation and the latest high tech equipment – notably a German made early model of the electrocardiogram. Regarding The Fitness Institute program, Percival stated, "It has not encountered one unfortunate experience in the five years it has been recovering cardiac patients." Percival re-iterated these claims on July 16, 1968, on the CBC television newsmagazine program, "The Fat of the Land."

1968 was also the year that Dr. Terry Kavanagh established his cardiac rehabilitation program at the Toronto Rehabilitation Centre. Considered the first of its kind in the world, it became a model for cardiac rehabilitation programs everywhere, and Dr. Kavanagh has quite rightly been showered with honours for his leadership in this field; however, it is clear that Percival began working with cardiac patients almost immediately after The Fitness Institute first opened its doors in 1963 and an effective program, which included regular medical consultations, was well-established before the opening of the Toronto Rehabilitation Centre.

The New Fitness Institute

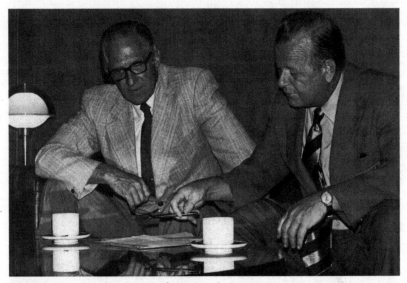

Jim Gairdner and Lloyd Percival signing their agreement to open a 'new' Fitness Institute in Willowdale in 1969.

AGE AND LIFESTYLE WERE CATCHING UP to the generation of successful post WWII businessmen of which the cardiac rehabilitation group was the thin edge of the wedge, and they were clamouring at the gates of The Fitness Institute. Percival also discovered that he enjoyed working with these men. Partly, it was a love of being in the spotlight that attracted him to working with the *crème de la crème* in any field. Percival also learned that, more often than not, these men were successful because they had achiever personalities. Athlete or businessman, dancer or musician, Percival loved to work with this kind of individual. In 1969, he and Jim Gairdner built a new home away from home for them. The new, bigger and better Fitness Institute occupied 4.5 acres of land at 255 Yorkland Boulevard in Willowdale, the north end of Toronto.

One-quarter of the memberships were made available to women, but in the early days of the new Fitness Institute, the vast majority of business people were still men. They were being informed by a medical profession that was becoming much more aware of health issues associated with lifestyle. On top of that, in the highly competitive world these middle aged businessmen inhabited, there was a wave of young executives eager to take their places. They couldn't afford to slow down. Percival said that he could make them younger, so they joined The Fitness Institute. He became a kind of pied piper for middle-aged businessmen, and plenty of younger executives tagged along.

John Wildman, who became president of The Fitness Institute when H.J. Heinz Company bought it from the Gairdner family after Percival died, liked to brag: "If a bomb were to go off in The Fitness Institute at eight in the morning, half of Canada's business elite would be wiped off of the face of the earth." Wildman was referring to a downtown location that didn't open until 1985, but the statement could just as easily be applied to the Willowdale Fitness Institute fifteen years earlier where many of "Canada's business elite" did their workout early in the morning before they jumped on the Don Valley Parkway and drove downtown to work. The *Toronto Star* proclaimed it, "The most dramatic example of the physical fitness phenomenon which is sweeping Metro (Toronto) and probably all of Canada."

If The Fitness Institute at the Inn on the Park was a fitness club with the trappings of a country club, the Willowdale club was the "Taj Mahal of health clubs." The combination of style and function that had made the original Fitness Institute such a success with both athletes and businessmen was taken to a whole new level in the Willowdale facility. Percival was not content to create the "most comprehensive conditioning and reconditioning organization in the world." His 1968 press release announced:

> The Fitness Institute will provide modern conditioning for the modern world. It will dispel health doubts. Remove apathy, and offer the key to a better enjoyment of life. It will improve the figure of the frustrated housewife, ease the tensions of the harassed businessman, build up the strength of the puny youngster, maximize the skills of the amateur and professional athlete, and rehabilitate those with medical limitations.

Chiselled above the doorway of the 50,000 square foot facility – ten times the size of the original Fitness Institute – was another of Percival's mottos, a quote from Hippocrates, the father of modern medicine: *Non Uti Est Abuti* which Percival translated as "No Use Is Abuse" or "Use It, Or You Lose It." Inside, male and female members enjoyed separate conditioning facilities including the first tartan running tracks in Canada. Few health clubs in Canada offered services for women at this time; if they did, hours and usage were restricted. At The Fitness Institute, women were able to use the facility whenever it was open and, for the most part, had access to the same state of the art equipment as the men. There were babysitting services available to make it easier for women to attend regularly, and the women shared with the men "the sumptuous lounge" with a colour television and an "ultra-modern restaurant."

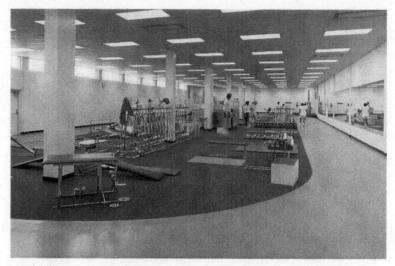

Men's Gymnasium and tartan track at Willowdale Fitness Institute.

There had been numerous improvements in testing equipment since 1962, and the new Fitness Institute had all of them including an area devoted solely to cardiac rehabilitation. Alan Scott, who joined The Fitness Institute shortly before the move, was a recent graduate of the University of Toronto Physical Education Program where he had studied under Dr. Roy Shepard, a renowned authority in health and physical activity and a pioneer in physiological research. Scott was teaching a fitness class at the Y.M.C.A. when one of his students, an architect working on the proposed Fitness Institute in Willowdale, asked him for advice regarding the testing facilities. This led to a meeting with Percival who sent him off to put together a proposal. Scott was familiar with the kind of equipment generally found in health clubs and universities; he had also seen the kind of equipment Dr. Sheppard had to beg and borrow from hospitals and university labs in order to do much of his seminal research. In addition, there was equipment that Scott had only read about such as the machine that NASA had developed for measuring oxygen uptake. He designed two fitness testing facilities for Percival. One was good and would probably have been the best such facility in Canada. It would cost $20,000.00. The other was a dream. It included anything and everything Scott could find to do the most in-depth and accurate testing of human physiology possible at that time and would cost $200,000.00. When he next sat down with Percival, Scott had both proposals in his briefcase, still unsure which he should present. Percival opened the meeting with the job offer Scott had been hoping for at which point Scott decided, "If I am going to work here, I'd rather work in a $200,000.00 lab." After Percival looked over the dream proposal – "only briefly" – Scott remembers him pronouncing "fantastic – we really need this – this is really going to make a difference in Canada."

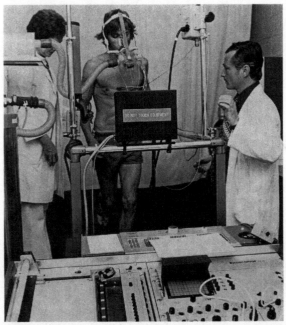

Prior to running 4,000 miles across Canada in 1974, Mark Kent, a 17 year old Toronto high school student, has his maximum oxygen uptake (VO_2) measured by Doreen Fraser and Dr. Frank Berka at the Testing Centre in the Willowdale Fitness Institute.

While the décor in the members' areas and the training rooms were intended to make the members feel pampered and comfortable, the testing rooms and medical facilities deliberately mimicked the scientific environment of a laboratory. In a feature article in *Maclean's*, Charles Taylor described them as "a cross between a hospital operating room and the torture chamber of an especially inventive sadist." Percival had the great fortune of finding Dr. Frank Berka working as an emergency room physician at Sunnybrook Hospital. Dr. Berka was a refugee from Czechoslovakia, an internist with a specialty in cardiology that was not recognized in Canada. Dr. Berka knew exactly how to use all of the specialized equipment that had been purchased and what equipment Percival still needed to make this the world class cardiology and high performance athletic testing centre that it was destined to become. Dr. Berka gave Percival's facility credibility. He was the link between the athletes and members and the scientific community that so often dismissed Percival

The Inn on the Park's seasonal recreation complex was replaced by all-weather, covered tennis courts, a 25 metre indoor Olympic standard pool with one and three metre diving towers, underwater windows and speakers, and an indoor golf complex. The golf enthusiasts who joined The Fitness Institute had access to driving cages with mirrors and cameras, putting and chipping areas, Canada's first Golf-o-tron, the prototype of today's computer generated indoor golf courses, video playback and computer swing analysis and a pro shop. Also new to the Willowdale location were squash courts, saunas, whirlpool baths and the latest in tanning rooms so that members would not only feel good, they would look good, too.

If there was ever any doubt that Gairdner would spare no expense to ensure that The Fitness Institute would be North America's most complete fitness and training facility, he proved it with the swimming pool. Designed to be up to Olympic standards so that any records set at swim meets would be internationally recognized, when the short-course pool was complete it was discovered that measurements had been taken without considering the inlay of tiles. Percival ordered the tiles removed and the pool rebuilt to proper specifications – The Fitness Institute never hosted a single swim meet.

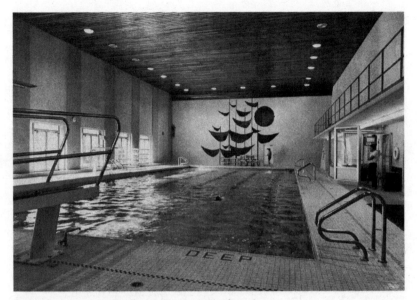

The 'Olympic standard', short course pool at the
Willowdale Fitness Institute.

There was an opening day staff of seventy, and each person had a university degree or the recognized equivalent; two-thirds of the staff were "technical experts." Soon after opening, the full-time nurse was joined by a full-time doctor. Percival also established a medical advisory committee, enhanced his already impressive library of international literature on sport and fitness – the Institute spent $5,000 per year to translate important articles in European journals into English – and built up a computer database of 70,000 individual case histories.

The service model Percival and MacLennan had devised for the Inn on the Park was ingrained in each new staff member. They were professionals serving professionals, and they were coaches. Scott and MacLennan became members of the American College of Sports Medicine and, along with selected staff, frequented conferences and seminars. All of the information garnered from these forays was presented to Percival whose ability to digest information never ceased to amaze those around him. Scott remembers how he would return from a conference late in the day or evening, drop thick volumes of research presentations on Percival's desk and be questioned on the minute detail of their contents the following morning.

Percival was known to all – staff, members, visitors – even to his daughter, Jan, simply as Coach. This title dated back to "Sports College" where he had been referred to as, "the head coach, Lloyd Percival." At the Inn on the Park, he was often addressed in this manner, but at the Willowdale Fitness Institute the title took on a noble bearing. Percival felt honoured by this form of address because he believed coaching, in its truest sense, was a most honourable profession. In 1969, he wrote a three page memo to the staff outlining what it meant to be a coach at The Fitness Institute. The memo elaborated on, but in no way departed from, this more straightforward memo he had delivered to his small staff at the Inn on the Park in 1963:

> Changing member's lives for the better is our mission. To do this you are to consider yourself as a coach, deeply and personally concerned with the improvement (physically and psychologically), of those in your charge ... Each member will be a challenge to you and you will be interested in meeting that challenge. Take deep and personal pride in your success.

The Fitness Institute was still proud to present this as a service model in 2004. By that time, professionally trained staff were readily available; in 1969, people with the appropriate training, as well as the kind of attitude required for the job, were difficult to find. Percival had happened upon a rich vein of talent when he hired Bob Bursach for the original Fitness Institute. Bursach was working at the front desk at a Vic Tanny's – having been promoted from cleaning the equipment – even though he had graduated from university in his native Yugoslavia with a degree in Physical Education and Biology along with a specialty in rehabilitating heart patients.

Percival took Bursach to the Inn on the Park in 1968 and doubled the paltry hourly wage he had been earning, eventually naming him head of the men's division at the Willowdale facility.

Bursach, as well as fellow Yugoslav émigré's Ivan Pintharic and Eddie Slogar, among others, were better trained than anyone coming out of a North American university. In addition, they recognized what a wonderful opportunity it was to work at The Fitness Institute and were willing to work long hours without complaint. While Percival was a very generous man and was never shy about reaching into his pocket to help someone out, he didn't really understand the monetary value of work. Even at The Fitness Institute, he never received the financial compensation one would expect for one of the world's leading authorities in his field, and his expectations of the appropriate workload for his staff corresponded to his personal workload. Doug MacLennan cannot recall a single time that Percival took a vacation in the eighteen years they worked together, save for his occasional weekends at Stoco Lake. Staff had to make a point of telling Percival that they needed time off or they would never get a vacation, and MacLennan recalls a time when he had been helping the Don Mills athletes at a track meet and reminded Percival that it was time for him to go and take his wife and new baby home from the hospital. Percival responded without thinking: "Tell her to take a taxi! I'll pay!" When MacLennan protested, Percival relented and, somewhat reluctantly, sent MacLennan on his way.

No matter what their goals, the men and women that joined The Fitness Institute received the full support of the dedicated staff. The person who arrived relatively fit and wished only to improve his or her ranking in the company squash ladder was treated the same as the Bay Street executive who had been told by his doctor that he wouldn't be around to enjoy all of that money he was making if he didn't shape up. Percival was just as proud of the difference he made in the lives of these individuals as he was of his efforts in helping athletes win international medals and always stressed that the best reason to get fit was to be able "to enjoy your vices more." There is no better example of this than Charles Kane, a semi-retired sixty-three year old businessman who said that he joined The Fitness Institute in 1971 because, "I got so weak that I couldn't tear the top off my favourite brand of scotch and I realized that I had to do something about my condition."

After three months at The Fitness Institute, Kane told *Executive Magazine*, "I've tightened up my diet on everything except booze, stuck to my exercises and lost 14 pounds. Don't have trouble with bottle tops anymore either."

Canada's "High Priest of Physical Fitness"

SHORTLY AFTER THE OPENING of the new Fitness Institute in 1969, Percival was honoured by the Ontario Government with the Ontario Achievement Award he had been denied in 1967. He was named to a committee of high-powered businessmen and politicians who were planning a domed sports stadium in North York, CTV asked him to prepare a scientific comparison of hockey players and figure skaters for its "Inquiry" program and he was, once again, a frequent guest on CBC television and radio programs. In the Toronto media, lifestyle and entertainment reporters competed with sportswriters for interviews. Lloyd and Dorothy were featured in an article on successful couples who work together; he was asked for his ideas on coping with the Christmas season, was caricatured alongside Sigmund Freud in a syndicated cartoon and was used as a point of reference in a review of a musical performance by Gladys Knight and the Pips. A few lines of Percival's poetry, under his nom de plume, Lou Allen, also appeared in the *Toronto Telegram*, and he was quoted by the media on everything from how to prepare for the annual charity "Miles for Millions" walk in Toronto, to menstruation and female athletes and how fitness leads to better sex and "marital well-being."

George Anthony of the *Toronto Telegram* gave Percival his most substantial forum in April 1970 when he produced a "Shape Up For Spring" feature that focused on television star Bruno Gerussi and his five week fitness program developed and supervised by Percival and The Fitness Institute staff. Every Saturday for six weeks, an entire page of the "Lifestyle Section" was devoted to Percival, Gerussi and numerous other celebrities who were engaging in fitness activities;

there were frequent updates and follow-up articles during the week. On April 6, the newspaper printed a copy of the program Percival had designed for Gerussi later reporting that they were overwhelmed with mail orders from people in Canada and the United States who had missed that particular issue. When it was over, Percival and Doug MacLennan hosted three, three-hour fitness seminars for readers who had become hooked on the program. Anthony reported that "the series was hotter than a pistol," and it was revived the following spring with Toronto media celebrities, Dini Petty and Wally Crouter.

The February 1971 issue of *Chatelaine Magazine* included an article on Percival and his "temple of fitness," advising the largely female readership "you don't get fit to be Miss Canada. You get fit to live your life more fully." For the price of a magazine, readers received an array of home exercises along with Percival's usual sage advice on the role of fitness in the enjoyment of life, including better sex, for which he made the analogy, "If you want to play good tennis you must play tennis regularly."

It had been a little over three years since the drug allegations had threatened to end his career. Athletes, coaches and administrators from as far away as India, the Soviet Union and Brazil toured The Fitness Institute and tried to copy it. It became a model for the world. Closer to home, George Anthony bowed down to "the exercise emperor," and Charles Taylor anointed Percival "Canada's high priest of physical fitness."

The Task Force Report on Sport for Canadians

THE CANADIAN GOVERNMENT'S OFFICIAL POSITION on sport and fitness changed dramatically during the 1960s, and this played a major role in Percival's emergence as Canada's fitness guru. After the initial excitement, Bill C-131 produced little in the way of tangible results in Canada's sportspeople. The broad brushstrokes used to draw it up and the generalities it contained provided a foundation for the eventual creation of effective government policy; but in the short term, there was only bureaucratic constipation. Of the total $25,000,000 that was available for the promotion of sport and fitness between 1961 and 1968, little more than $15,000,000 was released, and there was dissatisfaction over how it was allocated.

In the latter half of the 1960s, the dismal record of Canadian athletes at the Olympics and in international competitions and the widening gulf between the amateur hockey players representing Canada and those wearing the red jersey of the Soviet Union were becoming an embarrassment to Canadians. The fact that television sets were now in almost every Canadian home and sports coverage was both more extensive and more technologically advanced meant that this state of affairs was more and more difficult to ignore. At the same time, Canadians were experiencing a crisis of national identity that was both internal and federal, because of Quebec's "Quiet Revolution," and external and nationalistic, in terms of the country's relationship with the United States. These factors coalesced in a growing national awareness of the need for the federal government to become involved in the development and promotion of sport.

By 1968, Canadians had a new flag, a new National Anthem and a new Prime Minister, Pierre Trudeau. Trudeau's 1968 campaign platform included the promotion of sport as part of his cultural agenda and his speech in Selkirk, BC, had promised a "comprehensive inquiry into the needs of amateur sport." After the election, Trudeau made good on his promise. Newly appointed Minister of Health and Welfare, John Munro, quickly appointed Harold Rea, a Toronto business consultant, to chair the Task Force on Sports for Canadians. The Task Force committee also included Dr. Paul Winkle des Ruisseaux, a sports medicine specialist from Quebec City, and world champion skier and Olympic hero, Nancy Greene. Christopher Lang was appointed administrator.

The committee traveled across the country, holding open forums and "meeting with interested groups and individuals." In addition, commissioners visited Scandinavia and Russia to see their sport and recreation programs first hand and attended the Olympic Games in Mexico City where they met with Canadian athletes and officials. Twenty-five hundred questionnaires were also sent out to Canadian athletes, coaches and sports officials. Percival told Jim Vipond that he had not been sent a questionnaire, but that didn't stop him from submitting a twenty page document titled, Some *Suggested Procedures for the Improvement of Canadian Standards in Sport and Fitness*.

Public education emphasizing the inherent value of sport and fitness in Canadian society and the determination that coaching comes before all else are the cornerstones of this document. The creation of a coaches' association along with education programs for coaches and the structuring of coaching positions are discussed as well as the same kind of structure and education within the sports medicine, administrative and research fields. Since Canada's inability to defeat the Soviet Union in international hockey was a major reason for there being a Task Force, Percival called for amateur hockey officials to "shake off the traditional influences and methods and develop a new system" because "it is highly unlikely that the NHL will depart from their own system or give up willingly their own present influence, philosophy and purpose."

The other thoroughly modern aspect of Percival's submission is found in the understanding he shared with Marshall McLuhan of how electronic media was reshaping the way society functioned. McLuhan wrote in his most famous book, *The Medium is the Massage* (1967):

> Media, by altering the environment, evoke in us
> unique ratios of sense perception. The extension of
> any one sense alters the way we think and act – the
> way we perceive the world.

Percival concluded in his submission to the Task Force that the government should utilize the mediums of film and television for promoting sport and fitness because:

> The use of mass communication to upgrade all
> aspects of sports and fitness in Canada could
> produce an interest level, a motivational effect and
> an effective result that would take years to achieve
> if a more conventional approach was used.

Percival also echoed McLuhan's belief in the specific power of television wherein he added, "As we all know television is the most powerful of our modern communication media and accordingly, every effort should be made to use it to promote any sports development plan."

The members of the Task Force concluded their public hearings and finished collecting all of the submissions in short order. They produced fifty-four final recommendations; however, none of the committee members possessed the expertise required to transform the material into the kind of comprehensive document that Munro and Trudeau wanted to present to the public. Chris Lang recalls that when he discussed the problem with the Minister, Munro informed him that he "knew of a man who could do the job."

Douglas Fisher had not sought re-election in 1965 and was working in Ottawa as a journalist and lobbyist. He remembers a chance meeting with Munro on Parliament Hill one day in March 1969. During their conversation, Munro discussed his dissatisfaction with the progress of the Task Force and asked Fisher if he would be interested in writing the final report. Fisher asked if he could co-opt sports aficionado and Carlton University historian, Dr. Sidney Wise. Fisher and Wise then sat down with Munro's Deputy Minister of Health, Joe Willard, who sold them on the project. Within three weeks of Fisher and Wise being ensconced in adjacent offices and Lang running back and forth between the two, *The Report of the Task Force on Sport for Canadians* was complete.

With the recommendations of the committee already set, the main responsibility of Fisher and Wise was to provide the context; Fisher referred to it as the "justification." The justification, or framework, of *The Task Force Report* became an understanding of sport as culture which had its origins in Fisher's discussions with Lloyd Percival in 1953. Fisher remembered vividly their ruminations on time and the philosophy of Spanish philosopher, Ortega y Gasset. More importantly, Fisher remembered their discussions regarding the place of sport in Canadian culture and Percival's extreme disappointment with the *Massey Report*; "that it was too high faluten – old world – about Opera Houses and the like. There was nothing there about sport and recreation." When they sat down to write the *Report*, Fisher and Wise "translated a bit of Lloyd and his view that sport, technically, philosophically and theoretically merited equal attention with any other aspect of culture."

The *Report of the Task Force on Sport for Canadians* was released with much fanfare on May 12, 1969. CBC Television gave special coverage to the news conference and heralded the *Report* as "a crossroads in Canada." Harold Rea informed the assembled media:

> Sport is very important. We feel that Canada is way
> behind most countries in sport. There is a public

apathy to sport that worries us very much. We
think that it deserves to be elevated and should be
a much bigger part of our culture than it is at our
present time.

Unaware of his direct influence on this seminal document,
Percival had praised the members of the Task Force:

I think a great job has been done so far. ...They've brought a
fresh approach with some people who are willing to listen. I was glad
to see some people out of sport appointed to the Task Force rather
than the old administration with preconceived notions.

In the wake of the *Task Force Report*, the profile of sport in
Ottawa changed dramatically. A tidal wave of bureaucracy swept
over sport and fitness interest groups in Canada, and Fisher rode
the crest of the wave, quickly emerging as one of the most powerful
and influential people in Canadian sport and Percival's first important friend in Ottawa. Through Fisher, Percival became known to
a whole new group of bureaucrats and politicians. He also became
publicly acceptable to sports officials who had known him for years.
Together, they saw him as an ally in their campaign to transform the
fields on which Canadian sport and fitness were played.

The most significant of Percival's new friends was Minister of
Health and Welfare, John Munro. Munro recognized in Percival a
keen mind, a deep understanding and knowledge of sport and fitness
and, of great importance to a politician, a pipeline to the media and
popular opinion. Munro consulted with Percival often and the shape
and substance of sport policy developed during Munro's tenure as
Minister of Health and Welfare drastically and permanently altered
the way Canadians participated in and understood sport and fitness. Munro proved a very intelligent and effective promoter for the
modernization of sport in Canada, but he always remained an even
more effective politician.

Another important ally was Munro's Deputy Minister, Joe
Willard. By 1968, Willard was a seasoned bureaucrat. He continued

to have a strong belief in the role government could play in the promotion and administration of sport and, since 1961, had developed
an extensive knowledge of the inner workings of government. This
combination made him a critical asset to all of those who became
involved in profoundly changing the manner in which government
approached sport and fitness during this time, but he was especially helpful to Munro. Dan Pugliese, the first Co-ordinator of
the National Sport and Recreation Centre, says that Willard was
"probably the most important person behind the scenes" in the new
sports bureaucracy in Ottawa. He recalls how "Willard and I talked
to Percival many times, because he (Percival) was the first guy who
had the big picture – the management and technical sides."

The *Task Force Report* was an essential platform for a new government philosophy regarding sport, but it was the recommendations
contained within the 1970 document, *A Proposed Sports Policy for
Canadians*, which established that Canadian sport policy was finally
subjected to a rational and comprehensive approach. The *Proposed
Sports Policy* also ensured that the federal government recognized
the importance of associating sport with fitness and health for all
Canadians and, according to historian Douglas MacIntosh, this was
due to the efforts of "individuals such as Lloyd Percival (who) continued to preach the benefits of physical fitness for the health of
everyone in society."

The ink was barely dry on *A Proposed Sports Policy for Canadians*
when the International Olympic Committee (IOC) made an
announcement that brought tremendous pressure to bear upon the
nascent sports bureaucracy and the pivotal decisions that were still
being made regarding its shape and substance. When Montreal
mayor, Jean Drapeau, left for Amsterdam in May of 1970 to present Montreal's bid to host the 1976 Summer Olympics, few people
believed he had any chance of convincing the IOC to choose
Montreal over Los Angeles or Moscow. Drapeau's persuasive presentation which, given the legendary extravagance and residual debt left
by the 1976 Olympics, ironically featured the promise of a stripped

down "people's Games" convinced the majority of the IOC members. Drapeau returned home triumphant while Munro and his colleagues were forced to fast track policies geared to the improvement of Canadian athletic performance in international competition.

Lloyd Percival could not have been more pleased with these developments. He had been endeavouring since 1936 to convince the Canadian government that it should take a prominent role in the health, fitness and sporting endeavours of the nation. Now that the government was finally developing policy and the Montreal Olympics were providing a sense of urgency to their implementation, he was eager to play a part, and Munro obliged. Munro approached Percival in June and asked him to submit a brief "outlining what should be done to improve not only Canada's sports representatives, but the fitness of Canadians generally." Percival told the *Toronto Star*, "Munro struck me as being definitely determined to improve things, so I'm giving it one more whirl."

On September 1, Percival submitted to Munro a 200 page document titled:

An Evaluation:
Historical Background and
Recent Status of Sports and Fitness
Standards in Canada

Analysis of Present Programs
Available and Suggested
Amendments and Additions

The brief elaborates upon and provides more details to the 1969 submission to the *Task Force* – the discussion on hockey is omitted since it was being dealt with separately. It includes Percival's philosophy and historical analysis with a caveat that:

It has been said that to solve a problem successfully the problem must first be stated clearly so that its general nature can be clearly understood and an awareness developed of the detailed mechanics involved.

To that end, Percival's submission identifies structure, organization, levels of responsibility and coaching as the key weaknesses in the vast network of Canadian sports and fitness organizations. The lynchpins of Percival's plan were a National Coaches Association, a National Sport and Fitness Development Centre and National Weekly Television Program. Percival also pointed to a prevalent weakness in the development of Canadian sports that had been featured in many of his previous presentations but which was still a new concept to most Canadians in the field: promotion and marketing. Not surprisingly, the whole thing looks a lot like the plans for CASPFDS in 1956.

It is extremely important to establish that Percival did not present this brief to Munro as a litany of demands for government funded projects. He made general, as well as specific, recommendations regarding proposals for which private and corporate funding are necessary adjuncts to government subsidization, pointed out areas where private and corporate sources should be the primary financial support and suggested programs that had income producing potential.

Perhaps the most remarkable aspect of the *Task Force Report* and the steady stream of documents it inspired was the speed with which the government produced reports and responded to the recommendations. It was only five months after the formation of the Task Force that the commissioners released the report and even before the *Task Force Report* was tabled, it was being acted upon. Within seven months, action on eighty percent of the recommendations had been initiated, and *A Proposed Sport Policy for Canadians*, although tabled in the House in 1970, was never formally debated or ratified. It wasn't necessary; most of the recommendations were already in the process of being implemented.

Hockey Canada

URING A MEETING OF SPORTS CANADA in the mid-1970s, Marc Lalonde, John Munro's successor as Minister of Health and Welfare, was discussing the allocation of funds to various sports. As he ran down a long list of sports bodies that included hockey, Douglas Fisher interrupted him: "Pardon me, Mr. Minister, but in this country there is hockey and there is other sport, and the two should never be mixed-up." This simple statement helps us to understand the problems that amateur sports have traditionally experienced gaining public interest outside of Olympic years; it also speaks volumes about the passion Canadians feel for hockey and the problems this causes politicians in Ottawa. And it is the reason that more than one-half of the *Task Force Report for Canadians* was devoted to hockey and why the first arms-length agency to be created as a result of the *Task Force on Sport* was Hockey Canada.

Douglas Fisher was a member of the first Hockey Canada Board of Directors, appointed by Munro in 1969 and charged with making immediate changes to the way that amateur hockey was structured in Canada. Chris Lang was the Secretary-Treasurer. Fisher and Lang convinced the other board members, including NHL owners, David Molson and Stafford Smythe, to bring Percival on board to help Father David Bauer with the team of university students and NHL prospects Bauer was preparing for the World Hockey Championships in Winnipeg in March 1970. This was to be the first major international hockey tournament ever held in Canada and the first offensive for Hockey Canada. Fisher and Lang were convinced that Percival's knowledge of fitness and hockey-specific training was a weapon that Canada had neglected for too long. The appointment was a major breakthrough for Percival. It marked the first time that he had an official position with a national sports organization, and it granted him a tremendous opportunity to prove the efficacy of his hockey program.

Percival prepared another of his detailed and holistic training manuals. This forty-five page document was geared to counteract the particular brand of hockey played in Europe and contains a breakdown of the individual styles of the participating countries. The program covers the usual subjects: conditioning, total endurance, strength, tension control, diet along with a strong emphasis on testing to establish a baseline, to gauge progress and to measure the Canadians against known levels of fitness achieved by players from the other countries. Percival also framed his training manual as the first part of a more ambitious, long-term program.

In his summation, Percival was brimming with the excitement and anticipation he obviously brought to this project. He extoled the virtues of his program, even as a short term solution, and revealed something of the deeper meaning this opportunity held for him; the career validation he hoped it would bring:

> Recognize that though there is a long term
> plan involved, it is the coming World Hockey
> Tournament that matters right now and that if
> we succeed in our purpose (to win) we will not
> only give Hockey Canada (and Canadian hockey
> generally) a tremendous boost but we will show
> Canadian sport generally what can be done – we
> can show the way!

Players were tested at The Fitness Institute in the fall of 1969, and the team was given a new fitness program. Another battery of tests was scheduled at The Fitness Institute on January 5, 1970, after which Percival was planning to introduce phase two. The testing took place, but phase two was never required because on January 4, Hockey Canada announced that it had withdrawn the Canadian team from the 1970 World Hockey Championships due to a dispute over the proposed inclusion of professional players on the Canadian team.

Percival didn't agree with the decision, nor did he believe that it had been necessary for Canada to push for the inclusion of professionals in the World championships. He truly believed that in spite of what the Russians had accomplished using his ideas, they had not thought of everything. He told reporters:

> There is not a Russian alive who knows more about conditioning a team than I do. ... I'm not against NHL players representing Canada but I'm convinced we could have beaten Russia with the team we had. Now the points we had hoped to make may never be proved. Ah, if only things had worked out differently for once.

Percival later referred to the Hockey Canada decision as "the greatest single disappointment in my life," suggesting that Percival had expected to prove through the success of the National Team that everything he had been saying about hockey for decades was right. Because the success would have come at a world tournament held in Canada, officials from the whole spectrum of Canadian sports would finally have realized that there was another way of doing things – his way.

The National Sport and Recreation Centre

THE IDEA FOR A CENTRAL OFFICE to co-ordinate the activities of Canada's various sport groups was said to have been included in Percival's first proposal to government officials in 1936. He continued through the years to lobby for such an organization, often incorporating medical and other support services. As long as the government refused to get involved in the business of sport, there was little hope. When he created CASPFDS in 1956, Percival attempted to use "Sports College" to establish if not a geographical centre, at least a philosophical and operational one. In 1964, Minister of Health and Welfare, Judy Lamarsh, witnessed the disappointing performance of Canadians at the Winter Olympics in Innsbruck. On her return to Ottawa, she offered to build a national office for amateur sports. The government was willing to spend between two million and eight million dollars to build the complex in Toronto, Ottawa or Montreal. They offered to provide offices, meeting spaces and a library as well as professional and clerical staff. This was all to be done free of charge, and best of all, each organization would have been allowed to maintain its autonomy. Due to the weakness of the umbrella group, the Canadian Sports Federation, and the rampant paranoia within the various sports bodies, nothing happened and the administration of amateur sport in Canada remained a "kitchen table" operation. The 1969 *Task Force Report* made it a top priority to get Canadian sport administration off of the "kitchen tables" and into an administrative centre. Dan Pugliese, Assistant Athletic Director at Waterloo University before he moved to Ottawa to work with John Munro, was chosen to make it happen. Aided by corporate funding, Pugliese studied sports bureaucracies in other countries and took research teams to Sweden, Finland and Germany in order to help develop the entity they called The Administrative Centre. Pugliese also sat down on a number of occasions with Lloyd Percival because he knew "Percival to be the first person in Canada to push for the establishment of such a centre" and the one who best understood all of its ramifications. The first of the new breed of professional sports administrators moved to Ottawa in September 1970. In May of 1971, the new National Sport and Recreation Centre opened at 333 River Road in Vanier City on the outskirts of Ottawa. By 1978, there were fifty-seven sports and recreation associations in residence.

The Coaching Association of Canada

THE IDEA FOR A NATIONAL ASSOCIATION of Canadian coaches was the key component of Percival's proposal to the federal government in 1936, and all of his subsequent presentations to politicians included plans for some form of centrally directed, co-ordinated communication amongst the coaching fraternity in Canada. The political will to initiate policy in this area failed to materialize, and Percival's attempt to secure corporate funding for such an entity within CASPFDS was unsuccessful. Finally, with the publication of the *Task Force Report*, Percival could envisage the time when all of the coaches in Canada would be together under one umbrella.

Percival provided the details for his conception of a National Coaches Association in the brief he presented to John Munro in June 1970. He also outlined the qualities required of the future executive director of this association; under the heading "Possible Personnel," there was only one name: John Hudson. Hudson was a protégé and personal friend of Percival. He was also the only person in the country whose resume included local, national and international experience in coaching, administration and marketing. Douglas Fisher arranged for Percival and Hudson to meet with John Munro at the 1970 Commonwealth Games in Edinburgh to discuss the creation of a Coaches Association. Percival backed out at the last minute which brings up an interesting question regarding Percival.

Hudson was not surprised to find himself traveling to Edinburgh alone because he suspected that Percival had a fear of flying. While no one, including family, acknowledges such a phobia, there are only a couple of instances when people remember that Percival may have boarded an airplane. The globetrotting of his early years and his trip to the 1948 Olympics in London came before the advent of routine air travel and his passage on ocean liners was not unusual. Percival did not attend any Olympic Games nor any international sporting competitions that took place outside of Canada after 1948 in spite of his deep interest in these events. Curious incidents similar to Edinburgh include the 1952 Olympics in Helsinki when he made a last minute decision to stay home; frequent trips to Ottawa, Montreal and Vancouver for which he always chose to travel by automobile or train in spite of his busy schedule; and occasions when he was scheduled to deliver important presentations in Vancouver and New York, but at the last minute, sent Doug MacLennan in his stead.

Hudson met Munro for the first time in Edinburgh but came away with the feeling that the Minister was ready to move forward with the proposed association. Hudson followed up with at least three trips to Ottawa, and, in December 1970, John Munro formally announced the creation of the *National Coaches Association*. Of all the government initiatives in sport that are indebted to Lloyd Percival, the coaches association owes the most, and it is still referred to as "the brainchild of Lloyd Percival." However, after the years of dreaming, scheming and proposing, it took only a matter of months before his precocious off-spring proved to have a mind of its own.

It is not entirely clear what long-term role Percival expected to play in the coaching association. The legal papers establishing it as an "arm's length" government agency were signed in Ottawa by John Munro, on behalf of the Canadian Government and Jim Mossman, on behalf of the Association. Hudson was present but could not sign because he was going to be the executive director, a paid employee. Mossman, a member of the Board of Directors, recalls that he was asked to accompany Hudson and Percival to Ottawa because Percival was also disqualified from signing. Neither Hudson nor Mossman recall why Percival was unable to sign, and other Board members remain equally baffled. The logical explanation is that Percival was also expecting to be given some sort of staff position.

In the beginning, Percival did take on the unpaid advisory role of "Acting Technical Director" because the government was yet to fund the position of Technical Director in the various sports governing bodies. This role suited Percival perfectly. He had the position and de-facto authority but no actual accountability. His association with The Fitness Institute offered great satisfaction and allowed him to showcase his talents in a wide range of sport and fitness arenas. While it did not allow him the time to make the kind of full-time commitment required by any of the new sports bodies in Ottawa, history makes it clear that Jim Gairdner would have been more than pleased to have Percival act as a senior consultant and mentor to the young sports bureaucrats in Ottawa. Unfortunately, Percival was not prepared to slip quietly into that role.

Storm clouds moved in almost immediately, both figuratively and literally. After what Hudson describes as a very positive preliminary meeting in Ottawa in January 1971, Percival and Hudson, along with fellow director, Douglas Fisher and secretary to the Coaching Association, Christopher Lang, set off for Toronto in Fisher's car. Ottawa was in the midst of a horrendous snowstorm and all flights were cancelled. Since Lang and Fisher had to be in Toronto in the morning for a Hockey Canada meeting, the four men set out together on what turned into a seven hour drive during which Percival is said to have "resigned four or five times from the Association, over philosophical differences." The next day he delivered to the directors a thirty page letter full of anger and invective over the betrayal of his vision.

Percival's vision for the Association was one of a "gang of coaches – like Knights charging into battle." He did not want to begin by creating a bureaucracy. Fisher, Hudson and others believed that it was first necessary to build infrastructure because there were insufficiently trained coaches in Canada to lead the charge. Given Percival's constant complaining over the years regarding the coaching fraternity in Canada, it is surprising that he did not share this view. Much to Percival's dismay, the bureaucratic lobby won out.

Its victory was symbolized by a subtle change in the name of the new association, from Percival's first choice, the *Coaches Association of Canada* to the *Coaching Association of Canada* (CAC).

The first official meeting of the Board of Directors of the CAC was held at The Fitness Institute on February 7, 1971. At that meeting, Board Chairman Harold Rea announced that the first project to be undertaken by the *Association* would be a symposium on the Art and Science of Coaching. This had been a key component of the paper Percival had delivered to Munro a few months earlier, and Hudson remembers that allowing Percival to go ahead with this project so early in the life of the CAC was very much a peace offering from the Board of Directors.

Hudson locked horns with Percival on a number of occasions but believes that Percival was content to remain at The Fitness Institute and "run the CAC from afar." When government funding was finally announced and Hudson informed Percival that the CAC was going to hire a full-time Technical Director, Percival asked, "Why? You already have one." Hudson explained, seemingly to Percival's satisfaction, that the amount of work necessary to build the CAC and establish its credibility required a full-time staff person and that Percival's position as senior advisor would not be threatened; however, when Geoff Gowan was tapped as the first Technical Director of the CAC and Percival learned that Gowan would report directly to Hudson and the board rather than to him, Percival resigned.

Percival was not cut out to be a committee man. If he was not allowed to be in charge, he preferred to be somewhere else. This was probably an inherent personality trait intensified by his years in the wilderness fighting a lonely battle. By the 1970s, Percival had been fighting for so long and had become so set in his ways that he had difficulty listening to and co-operating with his peers. This inhibited his ability to play a continuing role in the CAC as well as in the burgeoning community of Canadian amateur sport. Still, the CAC and its sizeable impact on the development of coaches and athletes in Canada over the following four decades remains one of Lloyd Percival's greatest and most enduring legacies.

First International Symposium on the Art & Science of Coaching

Less than eight months after the CAC gave him the go ahead to organize the *First International Symposium on the Art & Science of Coaching*, Percival, Doug MacLennan, Joe Taylor and the rest of The Fitness Institute staff managed to organize an international conference that was without international precedent and has never been duplicated in Canada.

The *Toronto Star* described the forty man expert panel Percival assembled as "an athletic think-tank of outstanding depth." Canadians on the panel included: Dr. Roy Shephard of the University of Toronto; Dr. Gregory McKelvey of McMaster University; Dr. Michael Yuhasz of the University of Western Ontario; Dr. Max Avren, Senior Medical Officer of the COA; and Dr. Roger Jackson and Lou Lefaive of the Canadian Amateur Sports Directorate. Also present were John Hudson, Executive Director of the COA and some of the best coaches in Canada including national team coaches: Don Webb (diving); Lionel Pugh (track and field); Al Raine (skiing); Marilyn Savage (gymnastics); and Jim Mossman (canoeing). Canadian amateur and professional athletes were represented by Gordie Howe, Abby Hoffman, Al Balding, Nancy Robertson, Dick Shatto, Gary Cowan (Canadian Amateur Golf champion) and 1968 Olympic swimming silver medalist, Elaine Tanner Nahrgang.

It was the jaw-dropping list of international sports experts, however, which made this assemblage truly unique. Dr. James Counsilman of the University of Indiana and Forbes Carlile of Australia were the two best swim coaches in the world. Dr. Ernst Jokl, originally from South Africa, then at the University of Kentucky, and Dr. Per-Olaf Astrand of the Swedish College of Physical Education in Stockholm, Sweden were the world's leading sports physiologists.

Dr. George Dintiman of the Virginia Commonwealth University had inspired world-wide attention as both a coach and a sport scientist. Dr. Thomas Tutko of USC and Dr. Miroslav Vanek of the Charles University of Prague, Czechoslovakia, were recognized as the world's foremost authorities on sport psychology. And Dr. Bryant Cratty, Director of the Perpetual Learning Centre at UCLA, was recognized for cutting edge research where sport physiology and psychology were integrated. Percival said he was able to attract this diverse group of academics because the Symposium was to focus on practical application, not theoretical discussion. In Dr. Tutko's words: "The coaches are the people who have to apply the information ... and the gap in athletics today occurs between the appliers (coaches) and the people who actually participate – the athlete."

The *First International Symposium on the Art and Science of Coaching* was held at The Fitness Institute from October 1 through October 5, 1971. For five days, the 250 delegates – more than 200 applicants were turned down – attended presentations and panel discussions from 8:00 a.m. until 6:00 p.m. The topics ranged from the seemingly esoteric, "Values and limitations of muscular strength in achieving endurance fitness for sports," and "Psychological/physiological factors involved in recovery after training and competitive effort" to the more practical sounding, "The coach, his role and attitudes" and "Parent communication and training by the coach." It was an unparalleled success, "one of Percival's crowning achievements," and he was showered with praise from the experts who had participated. Dr. Jokl wrote to Percival after the conference was over: "I feel that you are the "bridge" between the scientist and the ordinary citizen young and old who should benefit from all that becomes known." Dr. Tutko referred to Percival as "a prophet in his own time" and stated:

> It was an honour to be part of such a meeting. I shall be grateful forever, considering it the highlight of my professional career. ... You have

been instrumental in creating sports history and are certainly due all of the recognition that accompanies that distinction.

And Dr. Vanek wrote from Prague:

I have participated in various scientific conferences in different countries, not only as a psychologist, but also as a member of the Managing Council of the International Society of Sports Psychologists, and I would like to say how very much I am impressed with this unique approach to an integrated type of symposium.

In 1973, Dr. Cratty demonstrated just how much respect for Percival had been engendered by the *Symposium* when he included Percival's Symposium presentation, "The coach, from the athlete's viewpoint," in his book, *Psychology in Contemporary Sport*. It is a rare distinction for a layman to have his research published by an academic of Dr. Cratty's standing, especially when included in a book that became a standard textbook for university courses throughout North America.

John Hudson believes that Percival was "striving to be academically accepted" through the Symposium and that its success provided him with a measure of personal vindication. The response from the international sports authorities in attendance certainly helped, but Percival continued to have difficulty gaining the respect of the Canadian academic community. When Dr. Shephard was asked what he remembered about the *Symposium* he replied, "The symposium seemed to be based as much on Lloyd's strong sense of intuition as a coach as on science as I perceived it, and thus did not appeal to me very much." This is in contrast to what Don Cherry said when asked "why the NHL never listened to Percival." "He was a college guy. When he mentioned the word scientific he was finished." It is one of the great ironies of Percival's life that professional sports people in Canada ignored him because they thought he was a "college guy" and too "scientific" while Canadian academics and sport scientists discounted him because he lacked academic credentials.

The complete *Proceedings of the First International Symposium on the Art and Science of Coaching* were printed and bound in a two-volume set by the publishing arm of The Fitness Institute, FI Productions. Douglas Fisher has referred to this publication as Percival's "magnum opus," and there is no question that the *International Symposium on the Art and Science of Coaching* and the publication of the *Proceedings* were landmarks in the history of Canadian sport. Unfortunately, not enough of the publications reached the coaching fraternity Percival had hoped to assist in Canada. The coaching community was not sufficiently evolved to utilize it, and because Percival was unable to work co-operatively, both the *Symposium* and the *Proceedings* were sentenced to obscurity. Like so many of Percival's contributions to Canadian sport, the *Symposium* was too far ahead of its time to be embraced by the community for which it had been created. In spite of the continued relevance of many of the presentations and discussions, history forgot about it very quickly.

The sports & fitness Instructor

M ANY OF PERCIVAL'S MOST SIGNIFICANT CONTRIBUTIONS to the understanding of sport and fitness in Canada during the "Sports College" era were made through "Sports College" publications. When he began feeling a little restless at The Fitness Institute and suggested a similar pipeline to the public, Jim Gairdner set up a publishing division, FI Productions. Joe Taylor, recently returned from Africa, became the senior editor and *Proceedings of the First International Symposium on the Art and Science of Coaching* (1971), the first publication. When Murray Koffler agreed to distribute a monthly tabloid through his Shoppers Drug Mart outlets, Taylor began editing the *sports & fitness Instructor* (SFI).

As a marketing arm of The Fitness Institute, *SFI* was never short on promotion for the facilities and programs, and Percival took full advantage of being his own publisher. Large swatches of the early issues were devoted to trumpeting his unique perspective on the upcoming 1972 Canada/Russia hockey series and afterwards to saying, "I told you so." Percival was also able to let everyone know about his predictions for the 1972 Olympics along with his ideas on how to improve Canada's chances in 1976, but SFI was much more than a marketing tool for The Fitness Institute and a vehicle for Percival's rants. It represented a serious attempt to provide tools for athletes and coaches as well as for individuals simply interested in improving quality of life.

The subtitle for the monthly publication was *A world of knowledge for the world of sport and fitness*, and each issue explored the same wide range of themes that had been the hallmark of "Sports College." Taylor and assistant editor, Paul Juhl, conducted interviews and wrote their own articles, as did members of The Fitness Institute staff including Doug MacLennan, Al Scott, Peter Elson and Alan Percival. Articles specifically targeted to women were contributed each month by the Women's Editor, Margaret Scott, who was succeeded by Esther Brooks and Roberta Picco (Angeloni). As he had with the *SCRG/SCN*, Percival disguised the extent of his own contribution by writing under pseudonyms Dorothy MacDonnell, Lou Allen and Alan Percival.

Articles appearing under the by-lines of experts such as Al Balding, George Knudson, Al Raine, Dr. Thomas Tutko, Dr. Miroslav Vanek and Dr. Bryant Cratty appeared on a regular basis and were heavily influenced by Percival. Sometimes, working with themes and ideas that were staples of these men, Percival would dictate notes or a rough draft to Taylor and Juhl, who then wrote the articles before vetting them with the named authors and applying their by-line. The fact that these experts, most of whom had international reputations to protect, trusted Percival and Taylor to work in this manner attests to the high regard in which Percival was held. That he was able to sit down and dictate from memory the advanced theories of the world's leading experts in sport psychology, physiology and coaching and was able to satisfy those experts with the authenticity of the writing is a testament to his encyclopaedic knowledge on a wide range of subjects.

As an example of how each issue of *SFI* included something for everyone from the new fitness convert to the aspiring athlete and from the community centre instructor to the national coach, the January 1973 issue included:

> A cover story on "What Makes Bobby Orr Great" by Alan Percival
>
> Lloyd Percival's regular page two editorial (for Jan. 1973 titled: "Sportsmanship")

Esther Brooks on exercises for woman's pectoral muscles

A column by Margaret Scott on proper eye care
Dorothy MacDonnell on nutrition
Peter Elson on stress and stress management

Lloyd Percival writing about energy and vitality

Dr. Tutko on communication between athletes and coaches

Hamilton Tiger Cats football coach, Jerry Williams, in the "Master Coach" feature

Lou Allen writing on hockey "secrets of scoring from a scramble"

The monthly "Coaching Award" presented to national gymnastics coach, Marilyn Savage

Lloyd Percival in conversation with Russian hockey coach Boris Mayarov

Canadian national basketball coach, Jack Donohue, on basketball

Peter Elson on isometric exercises

Tom Wells regular "training Room" feature on "Blisters"

National ski team coach Al Raine's article, "The Making of Champions"

"Agility exercises for curling"

A sports medicine article from Dr. W. Kerr

Lloyd Percival on exercises for the heart

A science corner feature on oxygen uptake

Fitness in the workplace

Relaxation exercises for bowling

Lest the reader conclude from the January 1973 example that the women's editors were only concerned with a traditional presentation of women, one needs only peruse a short list of topics presented by the women's editors to include "Your daughter the athlete" (June 1972), "Those Male Chauvinist Coaches" (November 1972), "The Myths of Menstruation" (March 1974), " Pregnant? No Need to Give up Your Sports Program" (July 1973), "Motherhood and the Athlete" (January 1974), and "Not Enough Incentive for the Older Athlete" (May 1974) to appreciate that Percival continued to espouse a very modern approach to fitness and sport for women.

The specific needs of children, whether or not they aspired to be athletes, were also targeted regularly. One article in particular struck a chord with readers at the time and has since become the most widely disseminated of all of Percival's writings. "How to establish rapport with your athletic child" appeared in two parts in the May 1973 (p.2) and June 1973 (p.2) issues. Percival credited Dorothy with the "ten commandments" he laid down, but it was Lloyd's constant search for solutions while others were busy complaining about problems that inspired the article. He had heard so many complaints about parents either being non-supportive of their athletic children or pushing them too hard that he discussed the issue with a number of young athletes, called on his years of experience and drew from his wife's wisdom for a list that would assist parents, the majority of whom he believed wanted to do the right thing but lacked the tools. This extremely thoughtful article has migrated all over North America, has been reprinted countless times and has been modified to suit particular client groups. It is even more relevant in the overcrowded and highly competitive world of youth sports today than it was when Percival wrote it, and it is currently posted, in its original form, on at least a dozen internet sites as diverse as the *Des Moines*

Register (newspaper), the (American) National Association of Golf Coaches and Educators Association, and the Luxemburg - Casco School District Basketball Booster Club of Wisconsin (the number of places where altered versions and imitations appear would be difficult to even estimate).

The *sports & fitness Instructor* enjoyed a brief life – June 1972 through September 1974. Those twenty-eight issues, however, represent the most comprehensive monthly sports journal ever produced in Canada and the only one intended for a mass market to give such a high profile to amateur sport.

ParticipACTION

MIDST "THE FLOOD OF DOCUMENTS" unleashed by the *Task Force Report* was a study commissioned by the National Advisory Council on Fitness and Amateur Sport (NACFA) supporting Percival's long-standing contention that Canadians were in terrible shape. In light of the study, Phillipe de Gaspe Beaubien, Chairman of the NACFA, convinced the government to provide seed money for an independent fitness promotion agency. ParticipACTION was incorporated in 1971, with Gaspe de Beubien as the President. The chairman of the Board of Directors was former Prime Minister, Lester B. Pearson; Lloyd Percival was a board member, and Lloyd Kisby was one of the first staff members hired.

In 1978, Kisby was named president and held that post until ParticipACTION ceased operations in 2001. He was also instrumental in the rebirth of the program in 2007. Kisby recalls meeting with Percival at The Fitness Institute during the planning stages but that Percival attended only one board meeting and did not contribute directly to the planning and development of ParticipACTION. It cannot be denied, however, that Percival contributed to the genesis of ParticipACTION. He had first outlined such an organization in his 1949 brief to the Massey Commission. In later years, he and De Beubien represented a two-pronged attack on government complacency regarding fitness and health that, if nothing else, softened the underbelly and weakened opposition to federal government involvement in matters long considered beyond its jurisdiction. When ParticipACTION became a reality, it couldn't help but look a great deal like a Lloyd Percival idea.

The marketing approach taken by de Beubien, Kisby and the board also bore Percival's stamp. As Kisby recalls, when they started "selling fitness like soap" the Board incurred the wrath of the university based "fitness professionals" who thought fitness was much too serious a subject to be presented in this manner. These were the same academics that repeatedly dismissed Percival as too "intuitive."

In the fall of 1973, ParticipACTION produced a fifteen second television advertisement that "changed the face of health promotion around the world" by suggesting that a thirty year old Canadian was only as fit as a sixty year old Swede. The commercial struck a nerve and probably did more to motivate Canadians to get off their couches and exercise than any other single pronouncement, program or event in Canadian history. Kisby developed the idea for the commercial after reading *Endurance Fitness*, a textbook written by Dr. Roy Shephard. In his book, Dr. Shephard quotes research studies relating to levels of physical fitness that he had carried out in Canada and Dr. Per-Olof Astrand had completed in Sweden but made no direct comparison between the two countries. Kisby and the advertising firm that produced the commercial drew the comparison in order to create an informative and entertaining product, intended to be more conceptual than factual. They did not expect the commercial to be taken literally and were surprised by the overwhelming response.

Percival claimed to be the source for the content of the commercial and had good reason for making the assumption. On April 15, 1972, the *Toronto Star* had featured the results of a four year study he and his Fitness Institute staff had carried out on "4,421 men and 1,675 women between the ages of 18 and 70 who had enrolled at his institute." Percival compared the results of his study with those previously published by Dr. Astrand. The newspaper included a graph of the two sets of results, under which was printed, "Canadian men aged 18 - 29 score the same as Swedish men 60 and over."

By the spring of 1974, Percival was probably aware that it was Kisby's imaginative use of statistics, not Percival's prescience that was the origin of the incredibly successful ParticipACTION campaign, but he was not above using the similarity of his study to the television advertisement to create a little publicity for himself and The Fitness Institute. He invited sixty-three year old Swedish businessman, Bjorn Kjellstrom, to the Institute for a battery of tests and arranged for the results to be published in a front page story in the *Globe and Mail's Weekend Magazine* on June 8, 1974, titled "It's True What They Say About Swedes." This article was a wonderful example of how Percival's egoism, vision and understanding of the power of the media so often worked to the benefit of all concerned. Although Percival knowingly, or unknowingly, misrepresented the facts and took credit for the Canadian research study behind the advertising campaign, ParticipACTION officials were not upset. Unlike the academics working in the field, Kisby and his associates were more interested in the success of their program than in their personal aggrandizement. They were not jealous of Percival's large following or the publicity he generated. In fact, they appreciated the interest and enthusiasm he brought to their work and recognized that this publicity stunt not only provided a great boost for Percival and The Fitness Institute but, because the focus of the article and the majority of its content was devoted to helping Canadians understand why this sixty-three year old Swede was so fit and what Canadians could do to emulate him, was a powerful promotional tool for ParticipACTION and its campaign to encourage physical fitness in Canada.

Canadian Olympic Association and Game Plan '76'

THE *TASK FORCE REPORT* HAD BEEN EXTREMELY CRITICAL of the Canadian Olympic Association (COA). The authors echoed many of the criticisms Percival had been levelling at the COA and its members since 1948 and set it as the prime example of everything that was wrong with sports governing bodies in Canada. To its credit, the COA responded by overhauling an organization that had been operating like an "old boys club" for far too long. One of the significant moves made by the COA, practically and symbolically, was to open the doors of the club to its long-time nemesis, Lloyd Percival. When the COA asked him for help in 1971, it must have given Percival a tremendous sense of satisfaction and validation.

In April 1972, William Cox, Vice President of the COA Communications Committee, asked Percival "to submit a Game Plan designed to prepare our entire Olympic team for the 1976 Montreal Games." With the support of Olympic Trust, the financial arm of the COA, Percival organized and chaired the Olympic Action-Decision Game Plan Conference at The Fitness Institute in early May. P.S. Ross and Partners prepared a synopsis of the resolutions passed at the conference in a report titled *Improving Canada's Olympic Performance: Challenge and Strategies* and presented it to the press on May 25. Key to the plan was a request for between five million and ten million dollars a year from the federal government. Cox advised that the COA needed to know within sixty days whether the government was going to act on the recommendations in order for Canadian athletes to be ready for the 1976 Olympics.

As predicted by Percival and many others, Canadian athletes fared poorly at the Olympics in Munich in 1972 winning a total of five medals – none of them gold. Cox and Percival refined their earlier report and on October 27, 1972, held a press conference at the Royal York Hotel in Toronto to announce *Game Plan '76':*

> Fabricated by Lloyd Percival from the musings of
> 35 experts and distilled over a period of a year into
> a unified purpose of the sports governing bodies, it
> has the aim of putting Canadian athletes into the
> top 10 nations in points standing at the Olympic
> Games in Montreal in 1976.

Cox announced that they had widespread support from provincial organizations and sport governing bodies as well as from CAC Executive Director, John Hudson. A number of corporate initiatives were noted to be in place to help out, but Cox put the onus back on the federal government, this time with an ultimatum:

> We want to lay it on the line right now. There is
> a moment of decision. If a crash program is not
> started right after the election, then we might as
> well relax as far as our athletes are concerned. We
> will have missed the boat.

The Canadian Olympic Association envisaged itself as the heart of this effort to prepare athletes for 1976, but its long-standing image as an elitist organization was problematic. When the federal government finally agreed to support *Game Plan*, it bypassed the work that Percival, Cox and the COA had been doing and, instead, adopted a plan formulated by a group led by Dr. Roger Jackson at Sports Canada. There is a certain irony in that it was Sports Canada, the kind of government body for which Percival had been lobbying for decades, and an organization that was being run by the new breed of sport bureaucrats that he had been instrumental in creating which usurped his role in the preparation of *Game Plan '76'* and relieved

Percival of all vestiges of his newfound influence in Ottawa. Jackson does not remember this as any kind of slight to his mentor. It is his belief that Percival was busy with Fitness Institute business at the time and had no interest in any continuing role with the new sport bureaucracy even though staff at The Fitness Institute thought that Percival was too busy with outside projects to supervise operations in Willowdale. It is one of the conundrums of Percival's last few years that no two people seem to agree on exactly where he wished to concentrate his energies and why he lost his influence in Ottawa. Perhaps this is because Percival himself was unsure. The "lone wolf" had been welcomed into the pack but couldn't figure out what he was supposed to do there.

There were a great many similarities in the two versions of *Game Plan*, and Percival had only a couple of points of disagreement with the plan that was adopted in 1973. One complaint was that it did not specify a concrete goal for the Canadian team. He believed that setting a goal for Canada to place among the top ten nations in point standing would push coaches and athletes to strive for excellence. This is the philosophy that Roger Jackson, as the driving force behind *Podium 2010*, would employ when he was setting the ultimate goal for the Canadian team to finish first at the Winter Olympics in Vancouver in 2010 and the philosophy he was forced to defend throughout the Games. In 1973, with only three years to prepare, Jackson and his committee chose not to put that kind of pressure on the athletes.

Individual Athletes and
Sports Organizations

THE NEW FITNESS INSTITUTE IN WILLOWDALE became a mecca for sports organizations and individual athletes from all over Canada. Those who had discovered Percival at the Inn on the Park continued their membership at the new location, and Percival was able to design even more elaborate and effective programming because of the sophistication of the new set-up. Al Balding and George Knudson had access to the most advanced indoor golf facility in the world. The technology built into the swimming pool allowed Jim Mossman to observe, and record for the first time, the underwater movement of the paddle and the boat through the water – technology that was also utilized by Hermann Kerckoff and his daughter, Claudia. And Peter Burwash could use the new technology and the year-round indoor tennis courts to upgrade his training program.

Sharing Percival's time was a legion of fresh converts representing more than twenty-five different sports including badminton, boxing, figure skating, diving, rowing, sailing, skiing, water-skiing, cycling, equestrian events, fencing, gymnastics, squash, volleyball, water polo, lacrosse, archery, sky diving and table tennis. Some looked to Percival to help them become world champions; others sought only a short-term fix or assistance in overcoming an injury, and there were those who were simply curious. All of them gained something from working with Percival, his highly trained staff and their state-of-the-art equipment. Many of these athletes and coaches left large footprints on the history of Canadian sport.

Percival and The Fitness Institute also continued to stretch the boundaries of physical training and how it contributed to all aspects of modern life. Canada's first Formula One race car driver, George Eaton, received a personal training program from Percival as did members of the National Ballet of Canada, and the cast of the hit musical, *Hair*. The RCMP also asked him to help prepare the Swat Team that was being assembled for the Montreal Olympics. Percival had finally convinced sports leaders in Canada that his methods were sound and was now helping individuals in other high-stress activities to understand how specific physical training could improve performance.

Figure Skating

In 1969, Val Bezic and his sister, Sandra, were Canadian National Novice Pairs figure skating Champions. Although still very young (Val was seventeen and Sandra thirteen), Val believed that they were ready to challenge the senior skaters. He also knew that he could use more upper body strength for the lifts and throws he was required to execute. Val tried a few different gyms in Toronto. At a "Gold's Gym type," Val looked around at the "big, muscle-bound guys" lifting barbells and at the list of four exercises he had been handed and knew he was in the wrong place. When he walked into The Fitness Institute in Willowdale and was introduced to Percival, he knew that he had found a home.

Val and Sandra became favoured pupils. Whether it was because Percival saw the opportunity to learn about and impact upon a sport that was new to him or whether it was the "drive and determination" that Val says he recognized in them, Percival took a deeply personal interest in their training. Sandra remembers "he really took us under his wing," opening early on Sunday morning just for them. After the workout, "he would personally do physio on us and then we would sit in his office for hours and he would talk to us about sport, fitness and training." They would go over diet and monitor everything in the program. The Bezics learned not only how to improve their bodies and minds through stretching and strengthening, diet and psychology, they learned why. The Bezics were probably the first in the world to do the demanding off-ice training that all skaters engage in today and are convinced that Percival's holistic program was a key to their success.

The Bezics' coach was Ellen Burka, a legend in Canadian figure skating. Burka was a very demanding coach. According to Val, her philosophy was "the more pain you could withstand, the more prepared you would be." The understanding of balance in training that Percival taught the Bezics was integral to their surviving the high physical demand of Burka's on-ice sessions. Knowing "that you cannot have maximum effort without maximum recovery" was central to their success and is something Val tries to instil in his children in their soccer training today.

Most doctors were of little help to athletes at this time. When confronted with a serious injury to a skater, doctors would typically suggest, "don't skate for six months." Percival's understanding of kinesiology and physiology still surpassed that of any coach in Canada, and his knowledge of where and how to access the best treatment for athletic injuries was a huge advantage for any athlete working with him. Frequently, this meant sending athletes to the United States. Percival helped Val Bezic find state-of-the-art diagnostics for a rotator cuff injury, designed the rehabilitation program and showed Val how to "avoid the impinging movements" that had caused the injury. On another occasion, when the pair was told that they were experiencing "a mental letdown," Percival correctly diagnosed anaemia and sent the siblings for blood tests. Val says today, "he taught me to explore everything and "this was a tremendous lesson."

Val and Sandra Bezic became Canadian Pairs Champions in 1970 and made their mark on the world stage. Unfortunately, Sandra suffered a serious ankle injury that ruined their chance for a medal in the 1976 Olympics, and they retired from amateur competition.

Val left the sport, unhappy that the cloistered world of figure skating was unable or unwilling to embrace the modern training techniques of Lloyd Percival. Sandra, on the other hand, introduced her own innovations to the sport. She became a renowned choreographer and the person who successfully married skating to television, producing more than twenty television specials as well as the successful series, "Battle of the Blades."

A few other Canadian figure skaters came to Percival for help including Toller Cranston, Lynn Nightingale and Karen Magnusson, but it was generally for injury rehabilitation. Cranston boasts of a body that didn't break down under the pressure of Coach Ellen Burka's demanding workouts and of being able to compete into his fifties without serious injury; however, he sought out Percival after suffering a groin injury in 1971. It was the day of competition. Cranston was unable to walk and "feared the worst." After Percival personally treated the injury, Cranston "walked out just fine." Cranston remembers being most impressed that, "The only thing that existed at that moment was to fix me."

Diving

Percival provided a home at The Fitness Institute to so many of Canada's finest athletes that it is hard to imagine the landscape of Canadian sports during that time without this facility. So many athletes and coaches remember the support provided by Percival and his staff, the way that staff understood the needs of world class athletes and the inspiration those athletes gained from training with other elite athletes from different disciplines. To athletes, the track, pool, weight room and massage table were like a second home. One coach went one step further and took up temporary residence in the parking lot.

Don Webb is a former professional high diving champion who became Canada's most successful diving coach of the 1960s and 1970s. By the end of the decade, his protégés included the two best divers in Canada, Beverly Boys and Nancy Robertson along with Cindy Shatto, a gifted young woman and daughter of Toronto Argonaut football star, Dick Shatto, and Scott Cranham, the best male Canadian diver of his generation. Dick Shatto was a friend and supporter of Percival and had introduced Webb to Percival. Percival happily opened up his facilities and resources to Webb and his divers free of charge. He also allocated pool time to Webb so that Webb could earn some money from teaching and helped arrange a coaching grant through Labatt's, without which Webb may not have been able to continue in the sport. After a short stint in 1970 as Technical Director of the Canadian Diving Association in Ottawa, Webb chose coaching over paperwork and returned to Toronto. While his wife was making arrangements to move the family, Webb lived in a camper in the corner of The Fitness Institute parking lot or, as the *Globe and Mail* described it, "Lloyd Percival's driveway."

Webb may have been the best diving coach in the country, but he quickly realized that his understanding of kinesiology paled beside Percival's. Up to this time, training for diving had consisted of hours at the pool doing dive after dive. Percival introduced a whole new regimen of nutrition, dry-land training and psychological preparation to Webb and his students. Webb says the "specificity (and) intricacy of what he (Percival) brought to the sport was more sophisticated than anything before." The divers were certainly aware of how much Percival had done for them. Of her time spent training regularly at The Fitness Institute, Beverly Boys says, "That was my best two years ever – we worked our asses off." Nancy Robertson remembers that "He helped us become more aware of our bodies and how to look after them." Percival helped the divers achieve a level of fitness that allowed them to just let go and "let the technique take over." They recall his calming influence, how he helped them believe in themselves and achieve a level of comfort on the platform, so essential in an event that is over in mere seconds. As Boys recalls, "he got into your head without getting into your head." After Boys won gold and Robertson a silver medal in their last event at the 1970

British Empire and Commonwealth Games (BECG) in Edinburgh, they sent a telegram to Percival:

> THANKS TO YOU AND THE INSTITUTE
> WE DID IT STOP WILL BE COMING
> HOME FAT GET READY STOP YOUR TWO
> SKINNYS
>
> BEV AND NANCY

Since Webb was the most successful diving coach in the country and his young divers were the core of the National Team for a decade, winning virtually all of the national titles and more than a dozen British Empire and Pan American Games medals (in the 1974 BECG, Canada swept the medals in the three-metre springboard event with Cindy Shatto upsetting second place Bev Boys and winning the gold medal), the coaching methods that Webb developed during his three year relationship with Percival and The Fitness Institute were widely emulated. He influenced a whole generation of diving coaches and administrators in Canada, including Boys and Robertson, who went on to distinguished careers in coaching and administration.

National Ski Team

Al Raine was named Head Coach of the National Ski Team in 1968 before being promoted to Program Director of Alpine Canada in 1973. One of his first acts in 1968 was to establish The Fitness Institute as a national testing centre for the ski team. Diane Gibson and Judy Crawford were familiar with Percival and his approach to training. Although Gibson's injuries kept her from fulfilling her potential, Crawford finished third in a World Cup in Switzerland in 1973 and just missed a medal when she finished fourth in the same event at the 1972 Olympics in Sapporo, Japan. The women's ski team also included Kathy Kreiner, who was only fourteen years old when she joined the national team in 1971. Although Kreiner spent much less time with Percival, she benefitted from the advanced training available at The Fitness Institute prior to winning four World Cup medals and a gold medal in the Giant Slalom at the 1976 Olympics in Innsbruck. While they may not have been aware of it, all of the women on the national team came under the influence of Lloyd Percival after coach Currie Chapman hired The Fitness Institute's Bill Gvoitch as a physical trainer.

The male skiers on the national team didn't have the benefit of a living legend like Nancy Greene to show them the way. It took a few more years for them to learn that they could compete with the Europeans who had dominated the sport for so long. Although Percival died before the glory years of the "Crazy Canucks" Ken Read, Dave Irwin, Steve Podborski, "Jungle" Jim Hunter and Dave Murray, he contributed to their success.

Jim Hunter was the first of the men to be influenced by Percival. Fitness expert Lee Coyne, who trained Hunter as a youngster as well as during Coyne's time with the National Ski Team in 1967, says that Hunter had always been "a radical" when it came to physical preparation. Working with Percival at The Fitness Institute in the early 1970s validated his intrinsic belief in pushing physical training to the limit and helped him win two World Cup medals. With the added confidence and credibility, Hunter believes he was able to push the rest of the Crazy Canucks to become fitter and, therefore better, ski racers than they would otherwise have been. He refers to Percival as "part of the chain in raising the bar for the team." Ken Read became the first North American to win a World Cup downhill ski race in 1975. He has acknowledged that Hunter "showed us how much work it took to succeed as a ski racer." Read has referred to Hunter as "the hare we all chased" and "the architect of much of much of our eventual success" while Steve Podborski remembers that the rest of the team "fed off of Jim's passion for hard work."

Podborski became the most successful of the Canadian downhillers but not until he became a regular at The Fitness Institute around the time of Percival's death. Even after Percival was gone, Podborski always knew that training at The Fitness Institute meant that he was training under Lloyd Percival. Podborski won twenty World Cup medals, one World Cup downhill title and a Bronze Medal in the downhill at the 1980 Olympics in Lake Placid New York. He might never have had the opportunity to shine if The Fitness Institute staff had not been there to ensure his complete recovery from serious knee injuries suffered in 1976 and 1978. Like so many other top athletes, the inspiration Podborski derived from the professional environment and the opportunity to train with many of Canada's best athletes was almost as important as the first class facilities and training programs. He says today, "I can't imagine what I would have done without it. ... It was fundamental to my success."

Podborski, Hunter and the rest of the Crazy Canucks were also provided with a competitive edge by The Fitness Institute research staff. Lee Coyne remembers that the men were having problems with "dead legs" at the end of the long downhill courses. Al Scott and his staff looked into this and found that the skiers' anaerobic capacity lasted only one minute to one and one-half minutes while courses such as the two classics, Kitzbuhl and Wengen, required more than two minutes to complete. Ken Read, who completed a rare "classic double" with victories on both courses in 1980, referred to Wengen's two and one-half minute run "as downhill's marathon" where "an extra thirty seconds on a very long run make racers vulnerable to fatigue and disaster." Scott designed "dynamic" weight training for the Canadian skiers that pushed back their "anaerobic threshold" and helped them stay strong right through to the finish. This contributed to the tremendous success of the Crazy Canucks at Kitzbuhl and Wengen.

The superb coaching from Al Raine and the other national ski coaches abetted by advanced physical training provided by Coyne, Percival and The Fitness Institute staff still may not have been enough had the Crazy Canucks not come to believe that they could defeat the legendary skiers of Austria, France and Switzerland. Coyne talks of the passion Percival helped instil in the skiers; Hunter remembers the motivational speeches that Percival gave to the ski team and the influence they had on him. According to Al Raine, "Percival's most important contribution was his focus on being the best in the world. For the men's team, this was a big leap at the time, however, only five years later the Crazy Canucks were world beaters."

Rowing

The St. Catherine's rowing club witnessed the success of the local schoolboy rowers who had implemented Percival's training program in 1965 and began using it themselves. One of the St. Catherine's rowers was Neil Campbell, who had represented Canada at the 1964 and 1968 Olympics. After retiring as a competitor, Campbell became the coach at Ridley College, a private boy's school in St. Catherine's. One of his first acts was to call up Lloyd Percival. Their collaboration was so successful that, by 1973, the Ridley College Eight had won four of six Canadian Schoolboy Championships, four straight U.S. titles and the 1970 and 1973 Royal Henley in England – victory was denied in 1972 when they crossed the line first but were missing a crew member who had fallen out. They were so dominant that after winning by five lengths in 1973, some of the Henley officials argued that they did not belong in the schoolboy race.

Campbell has stated:

> The best thing I ever did was go to see Lloyd at The Fitness Institute. ... We set up a continuing program of testing, off and on water conditioning and general consultations. ...We not only discuss training methods and competitive problems from both psychological and physiological viewpoints but he motivates (the) heck out of me.

Cycling

For many years, Percival had promoted the virtues of cycling as a form of fitness training. The Fitness Institute was a pioneer in the use of exercise bicycles in training programs for competitors in all sports and, in the early 1960s, Percival worked with the Canada Cycle and Motor Company (CCM) in designing the first stationary bicycles for home use (the home rowing machine they also developed together would not catch on for more than a decade). Percival also believed that riding a real bicycle was even more beneficial to the recreational athlete because it involved communing with one's environment and, in 1972, he wrote a foreword for *The Canadian Bicycle Book*. Only after Jocelyn Lovell and Peter Penman came to The Fitness Institute in 1969 did Percival introduce his special brand of training to the world of competitive cycling. By this time, Lovell was well on his way to gaining the same kind of reputation within the Canadian cycling community that Percival had long held throughout the world of Canadian amateur sports – that of a rebel who loved to thumb his nose at people in authority and always demanded the freedom to do things his own way. Perhaps this is why the two men got along so well. Lovell was self-taught and says that he never had a coach, but he was referred to as one of the "most intelligent men in the cycling world" because of his ability to look, listen and absorb. While he credits Percival with some of the innovations in his training program such as the weight training that helped him as a competitor, it is in more subtle and psychological ways that Percival made the biggest contribution to his success.

Lovell was another elite athlete who thrived in the presence of so many other serious athletes at The Fitness Institute. Being around Percival and the other elite athletes, he says today that one could "learn from osmosis." Lovell would bring new training ideas to Percival who would help him incorporate them into his program. Percival inspired him to approach his sport "from a thinking, scientific point of view," and was instrumental in Lovell learning that "the mind can control your thoughts" and allow you to do things in sport that you never thought possible.

Lovell was Canada's dominant cyclist during the 1970s. He won forty-one national titles, a slew of Pan-Am Games medals, more

British Empire Games medals than any cyclist in history, a silver medal at the 1978 World Championships but was deprived of his best shot at an Olympic medal by the 1980 boycott. Lovell was Canada's Athlete of the Year in 1975 and is credited with resurrecting the sport of cycling in Canada. After one of his medal winning rides in the 1970 Commonwealth Games, Percival sent a telegram congratulating the cyclist. Lovell's response read:

> Dear Coach:
>
> I got your telegram the day after my ride. Thanks.
> You know you own a piece of that medal.

While training near his home in Milton, Ontario, in 1983, Jocelyn Lovell was hit by a truck and suffered serious spinal cord damage. Within a couple of years, the fiery temperament that had gained him the nickname "the bad boy of cycling" was focused on the medical community and its failure to devote enough resources to finding a cure for spinal cord injuries. Today, he remains a leader in that fight and an outspoken advocate for spinal cord research.

Individual Athletes

George Athans Jr. was seventeen years old, born into one of the royal families of Canadian sports, and already a Canadian National Senior Waterskiing Champion when he arrived at The Fitness Institute in 1969. Younger brothers, Greg and Gary, both won numerous championships inside and outside of Canada skiing on snow and on water. George Jr. also excelled on the snow but turned down an opportunity to join the national ski team. George Jr. says that he and his brothers were "blessed with natural talent" inherited from their father, George Athans Sr., who first represented Canada in diving at the 1936 Olympics when he was only fifteen years old and finished seventh at the 1948 Olympics. It was George Jr. who took that natural talent and pushed himself the furthest. Although he retired when he was only twenty-three years of age, Athans Jr. won thirty-three national titles, four consecutive World Championships (1971 to 1975), was honoured as Quebec's athlete of the decade, named a member of the Order of Canada and became half of the first father/son combination inducted into the Canadian Olympic Hall of Fame. Perhaps that little bit extra came from his training at The Fitness Institute.

Officials in the waterskiing federation had the foresight to send Athans Jr. to Percival because he was still a teenager and they felt he "could use a little muscle." Of course, he got much more. Percival designed a nutrition program for Athans Jr. as well as weight training and circuit training programs specifically tailored to the needs of his sport. Athans Jr. believes that these programs were crucial to his improvement because he was competing against Americans who were able to spend twelve months of the year on the water while in Canada, he was limited to six. In a training manual that he later wrote for all water skiers, Percival argued that the training program developed for Athans Jr. which combined six months of training on the water with six months of dry-land training was superior to the traditional year-round on-the-water program.

Bob Domik was already one of the best softball pitchers in Canada before he hooked up with Lloyd Percival, but it was after he spent time at The Fitness Institute that Domik led the Richmond Hill Dynes to victory in the 1972 World Softball Championships. Domik didn't give up a single earned run in his four victories and was named "best pitcher in the tournament." He credited "a special arm-conditioning program" designed to "add strength, flexibility and power to the pitching arm" and to "keep the pitcher free from muscular tension." Domik's story was included in a page devoted to training for baseball in the June 1972 issue of SFI. After receiving requests from all over North America for copies of the "ten point program" Percival had designed for Domik, it was published in the July 1973 edition. The Toronto Maple Leafs Baseball Team was sufficiently impressed to do what their hockey playing namesake never did – hire Lloyd Percival to design a training program for the entire team.

Leo Cahill was hired to coach the Toronto Argonaut Football Team in 1968. He had been in town for a few years coaching the Toronto Rifles of the Continental Football League and was familiar with the reputation of Lloyd Percival. In 1969, he began sending his players to The Fitness Institute in Willowdale for rehabilitation, and Cahill himself received treatment from Percival. Perennial all-stars Dave Raimey and Jim Corrigal spent a lot of time there, and Charlie Bray became so comfortable at The Fitness Institute that Percival gave him a job in the off-season. In response to Bray asking what he could pursue in his spare time, Percival told him "anything you want." Bray began studying sumo wrestling and now runs a highly successful program for inner-city children in Buffalo, New York, called "Sumo Kids."

The story of Debbie Van Kiekebelt's time training with Percival is not one of glory and success, but it is instructive. Van Kiekebelt was an eighteen year old high school student when she entered the 1972 Olympics in Munich. She was ranked fifth in the world in the pentathlon and was one of Canada's best hopes for a medal. Van Kiekebelt failed to live up to anyone's expectations, including her own, and returned home "completely disheartened" and disenchanted with track and field.

Van Kiekebelt had come to Toronto from Calgary in 1970 in order to train with John Hudson's Scarborough Track Club. Hudson put her in the capable hands of Walter Kostric, another of the superior technical coaches who had immigrated to Canada from the former Yugoslavia. With Kostric's help, Van Kiekebelt quickly gained proficiency in all five events that make up the gruelling pentathlon; however, Kostric was the kind of coach Percival identified by the title "critic" in the classification of coaches he presented at the *Symposium*. No matter how successful she was, Kostric made Van Kiekebelt feel that she wasn't performing well enough. In his *Symposium* presentation, Percival argued that by constantly criticizing the athlete and not accentuating the positive, this kind of coach "makes the athlete feel that (she) never does anything right" even though "there are times when (she) just wants approval." A couple of months after her return from Munich, John Hudson convinced Van Kiekebelt to talk to Percival, and he agreed to take over her coaching. All parties concerned thought that this was a great opportunity for both coach and athlete. Van Kiekebelt loved working with Percival because she says, "he made you feel like you were the greatest." After just six weeks with Percival, she had her confidence back and was enjoying track and field again. A victory at a major meet in Montreal over a field that included the Russian woman who had finished fourth in Munich confirmed that she was on the right path. Unfortunately, Percival was not supplying a level of technical support commensurate to the psychological assistance she was receiving.

Van Kiekebelt and Kostric had spent two years working together on the track for as many as five hours a day; with Percival, she was getting only a couple of afternoons in his office each week. This was frustrating because she knew from conversations with former Don Mills athletes that Percival was an excellent technical coach. He just didn't have enough time for her. With all of the other projects he was involved with in 1973 and the stream of people who showed up at his door now that he was a celebrity, Percival could not be the kind of personal coach Van Kiekebelt needed. After a year, she reluctantly told him that she was going to seek coaching elsewhere. Like Jackie MacDonald in 1955, Van Kiekebelt didn't find that coach and never reached her full potential. She remembers that Percival felt badly for not being able to come through for her and laments that she did not work with Percival when he was a dedicated track and field coach.

The Cast of Hair

Due to the celebrity status enjoyed by Percival and his Fitness Institute, senior executives, politicians, actors and all manner of famous people were known to call him up and ask for a consultation. Percival almost always took care of these celebrities himself behind closed doors, although, depending on the problem and the nature of the intervention required, a trusted staff member might be assigned to do some therapy in private. One such visitor was Michael Butler, wealthy polo player and producer of *Hair*, the ground-breaking theatrical production that took New York by storm in 1967 before becoming a worldwide phenomenon. The Toronto production was mounted in 1969, and Butler became a frequent visitor to the city. During one of those visits, he was referred to Percival because of a problem with his arm. Butler was so impressed with the treatment he received and the facilities he toured that he contracted The Fitness Institute to do something about the rash of injuries that plagued the Toronto cast.

It didn't take long for Percival to diagnose the problem. *Hair* was a physically demanding show. It contained almost three times the number of musical numbers found in a traditional Broadway show, and many of these required a great deal of athleticism. Even trained Broadway performers would have found the show challenging. But the very nature of *Hair* and its celebration of "hippie culture" meant that most of the actors were untrained in the rigours of dance and how to prepare their bodies for eight shows a week. Percival introduced a stretching regimen for the actors to do before rehearsal and evening performances.

Percival and his staff also realized that the lifestyle of the actors was a contributing factor. They arrived for their evening performance without having eaten properly; after the show, they would devour something unhealthy like a burger and fries before partying into the wee hours and indulging in their drug of choice. The following day, they would appear at rehearsal, again, without having eaten properly. Percival told Butler that it was essential that they improve the nutritional intake of the performers. A buffet was laid out for the cast two hours before rehearsal, two hours before the show and immediately after the show. Percival had no control over how the cast members took care of their bodies the rest of the time, but the stretching and the meals ensured that the cast members were physically and nutritionally better prepared for the demands of their jobs and less likely to be injured. Butler was so impressed with the results that he had a home fitness program devised for himself, and Doug MacLennan flew to Chicago to instruct Butler's valet in how to administer it. In addition, The Fitness Institute was contracted to replicate their work with the Toronto cast for *Hair* productions in New York, Chicago, Boston, Miami, Hawaii and Las Vegas. Al Scott was in Las Vegas to do the initial fitness tests on the local cast when all of the male cast members arrived dressed in drag. This was the Vietnam War era when young American males were subject to the military draft. They thought it was a trick, and the fitness tests were actually being conducted by the draft board. The young men were doing their best to make themselves unfit for military service.

Percival loved his continuing work with the Toronto cast just as he always enjoyed young people who had a sense of vitality, and the staff enjoyed the break from their usual routine; however, even Percival's chain-smoking couldn't prepare the membership for the smell of marijuana wafting through The Fitness Institute lobby, and some of the corporate business men may never have recovered from the sight of young women parading around topless.

Hockey

B Y 1972, PERCIVAL'S METHODS had gained sufficient credibility within the NHL, or perhaps it was more that the players and their new union had acquired sufficient freedom from their overlords so that the players no longer had to don disguises before entering The Fitness Institute. The St. Louis Blues, Philadelphia Flyers and Detroit Red Wings even encouraged players to visit Percival, and a total of ninety-four current NHL players and draft choices worked out at The Fitness Institute prior to the 1972 season. In addition, Head of Officials for the NHL, Scotty Morrison, sent all of the NHL referees and linesmen to The Fitness Institute for testing and a training program. The biggest news in hockey that year was the announcement of an eight-game series to be contested by the National Team of the Soviet Union and an NHL all-star team. The series forever changed the way Canadians understand hockey, and, although he had no direct role in the events which unfolded, the landmark series helped to expose Percival's extraordinary contribution to the game of hockey as well as the woeful neglect he had suffered at the hands of Canadian hockey officials.

The 1972 Canada/Russia Summit Series

"It was obviously our way of life against theirs. ...
It was freedom against communism."

PAUL HENDERSON.

In 1972, Canadians combatted the evil forces of communism not on a battlefield but in the secular place that Canadians hold most sacred – the hockey arena. On the afternoon of the final game in Moscow:

"Factories stopped producing, schools wheeled TV's into class-rooms and Parliament stopped arguing. ... It is believed that three of every four Canadians were either listening or watching." Due to the political and ideological implications, Paul Henderson's winning goal became the one historical event that Canadians remember above all else. As McLuhan informs us, it was "their first vivid experience of national identity."

Lost in the emotional fallout from the Summit Series is the fact that the Canada-Russia confrontation began with a great deal of anticipation given the clash of ideologies but with no expectation of the high drama that the hockey was to provide. In spite of eighteen years of escalating concerns over Russian incursions into Canada's game, only a brave few publicly acknowledged that the Russians had a legitimate chance to win the series. *Montreal Star* reporter, John Robertson, was convinced that the timing of the series played right into the hands of the Russians. Billy Harris, who had coached Sweden in the 1972 World Championships, thought that Vladislav Tretiak might steal the series, and Lloyd Percival asserted that Canada would prevail only "if we do all the intelligent and very necessary things to prepare for this confrontation. ... If we are cocky or prepare casually, it's six to five either way and I wouldn't bet a nickel," he pronounced.

Percival knew more about Russian hockey than anyone else in Canada, and he was more than willing to share his knowledge. He had met with Tarasov and a number of other Soviet coaches and officials during the 1960s and had studied their games and kept statistics on all of the national team players. He understood their training methods because they were the same as his. Like every egotistical coach, he believed that he knew something that the other coach, in this case Tarasov, didn't know. This is what he had hoped to prove with Team Canada in 1970. In 1972, he had no official role and was limited to offering advice on short term preparation.

In the inaugural issue of the *sports & fitness Instructor* published in June 1972, he offered a plan. First there needed to be a "thorough, realistic evaluation of the opposition. … Every film available, every player and coach who has competed against the Russians, every observer who has analyzed them, must be tapped for a contribution." The players should be "prepared to start a scientific conditioning program at least six weeks before the schedule starts and one month before getting on the ice as a team." Percival demanded the best medical and training care for the players and advised that the team should be selected for "their poise, dedication to 'win for Canada' and proven adaptability as well as their excellent frustration tolerance." In light of the short preparation time, team compatibility was stressed over individual skill when selecting players, and psychological preparation was to be a top priority.

During the summer coaches were chosen, a team was selected and Alan Eagleson emerged as the de-facto commander-in-chief of all Team Canada operations. Percival offered the facilities at The Fitness Institute as a training base as well as his personal services. He wrote to Team Canada Head Coach, Harry Sinden, on three separate occasions without receiving a reply. Sinden later acknowledged receiving the letters but explained that he was getting "advice from so many people, it was swamping us." Douglas Fisher, Chairman of Hockey Canada at the time, remembered Sinden and assistant coach, John Ferguson being more blunt when he and others suggested that they seek help from those who had played and coached against the Russians: "We were told with some disdain to 'Leave it to the pros' or 'Don't burden us with bushers.' " Percival later surmised, "Maybe because everyone was so sure Team Canada was going to wipe out the Russians, no one wanted to share the glory."

More than thirty years later Sinden confirmed Percival's suspicions by stating, "The people involved were not going to let anyone else in on what was going to be an easy victory."

Sinden showed the players only three short films of the Russians playing hockey – one film was vintage footage of his 1958 Whitby Dunlops playing the Russians which reminded the players more of the Keystone Cops than of serious hockey. There was none of the dry land training Percival prescribed for the Canadian players, and on-ice workouts began three weeks before the first game was scheduled to be played in Montreal, instead of the six weeks Percival said was necessary. Sinden later attested that many of the drills he used for the training camp had come from Percival's *The Hockey Handbook*, and he is undoubtedly correct in stating that the players would not have agreed to participate in a six week training camp. But his statement to the *Montreal Gazette* prior to the start of the Series, "All I know for sure is that I don't want us to do anything that the Russians do," reveals how Sinden and everyone else associated with the Canadian team were completely out of touch with the state of hockey outside of the NHL. After seventeen days, Ferguson told Sinden that "It's as good as any training camp I was ever at with Montreal." Sinden agreed that "It was one of the most rigorous programs I led as a coach." Once again, "good enough" was considered "good enough" for Canadian hockey

Much of the second issue of *SFI* was devoted to Percival's views on the upcoming series. He lamented the late start of training camp and the nature of Canada's preparation but still hoped that the series would help Canadians – and perhaps even Team Canada if they bothered to read it – to understand what the Canadian players were up against and how the series was likely to unfold. Percival also outlined the "secret game plan" of Russian coach, Anatoly Tarasov. In spite of Tarasov having been replaced behind the bench by Victor Bobrov, the series would still hinge on decades of Tarasov's philosophy and coaching style. According to Tarasov:

> It is my view that collective effort, if it is performed
> with skill, will always defeat individual effort
> regardless of its brilliance, though perhaps it would
> be a battle to live on in your sports history since
> your NHL professionals are truly magnificent in
> their adeptness at least when on the offensive.

The "battle" does live on in our history because of the individual brilliance of the Canadians and because of the Tarasov approach which Percival correctly predicted would depend on constant attacking pressure, an unrelenting high tempo, a physical and psychological preparation that would stand up to Canada's attempts to physically intimidate, quick counterattacks, the use of numerical superiority in the attacking zone, quick passing, constantly changing patterns of attack and the use of brains over brawn. Percival's 3,000 word article contains much more detail on Tarasov's brand of hockey as well as Percival's suggestions on how Team Canada should have responded to it. The article was reprinted, in its entirety, in the *Globe and Mail* on August 19 and in an altered form in the September 2 *Toronto Sun Special Edition* devoted entirely to the Summit Series. For anyone who read one of these articles, the way the Soviets dominated the first game in Montreal on September 2, should have come as no surprise, including Sinden who had used the Toronto Sun articles by Percival to motivate the players.

The September issue of *SFI* also includes "Things you always wanted to know about Russian hockey (but didn't know who to ask)," p.11. Percival's most original contribution to the analysis of the Canada/Russia confrontation, however, appeared here as a comparison of the two teams based on his Sports Power Index. This was a complex rating system born out of the less sophisticated statistical analysis Percival had used for his 1951 comparison of Gordie Howe and Rocket Richard. It allowed "Sports College" to "evaluate the relative importance of the various performance factors involved in any game or event." Through scientific measurement, the various factors involved in winning a hockey series of this magnitude were determined, and the teams were scored in each of twenty-nine weighted categories. According to Percival's scoring, Team Canada possessed a decided edge in the skill categories while the Russians were physically superior by a wide margin. When totalled, Team Canada earned 2,388 points compared to 2,383 points for the Russians (even this small difference evaporates when you note that

Gary Mossman

Percival badly underestimated the value of Tretiak in goal). Percival also discussed some of the individual findings of his Sports Power Index. In particular, he presented his case for the importance of maximum oxygen uptake (VO2) in comparing aerobic endurance. While this is old hat for sports testing today, as it was for Percival then, it was something professional hockey knew nothing about in 1972. Percival had acquired test results for the Russian players which revealed an average score of 75, a very good score for an athlete in a sport such as hockey (a VO2 score of 85-90 is still considered exceptional). From tests he had done on hundreds of NHL players over the years – some of who were with Team Canada – he estimated the Canadian team would achieve 53.5 as the score if tested as a group.

In a footnote to the *Toronto Sun* article, Percival pointed out that Paul Henderson's score of 67 was the highest recorded by any Canadian hockey player he had ever tested. Percival concluded, "His (Henderson's) skating endurance and sustained speed show the advantage of having a good rating." The Canadian coaches did not expect Henderson to be one of the stars of the team, but his performance in the series, particularly during the latter stages of the last few games, underscores the validity of Percival's scientific approach. For some reason, Percival did not take credit for Henderson having achieved this high level of fitness through his eighteen months of training at The Fitness Institute. It is also interesting to note that the Russian scouts, Chernychev and Kulagin, told Percival, just days prior to the first game, that the two Canadian players who most impressed them were the men who would emerge as Canada's heroes: Phil Esposito for his "hockey thinking" and Henderson "for his speed."

Esposito and Henderson's dramatic rescue effectively wiped the memory of the previous seven games from the collective consciousness of Canadian hockey fans. The threat to Canada's game, which reverberated from coast to coast during the Canadian leg of the series, was so dramatically diffused by the last-minute victory in Moscow, and the effect was so cathartic, that Canadian hockey soon

302

reclaimed its smug complacency. The Russian demonstration of skill, strength, speed, fitness and poise, which probably would have resulted in victory if Tarasov had been behind the Russian bench, should have acted as a wake-up call for coaches and administrators at all levels of hockey in Canada. Instead, it was overwhelmed by the celebration of Canadian grit and determination, the glorification of the virtues of free enterprise and our democratic way of life. Canadians decided that the Russians had demonstrated "a different way of playing hockey, not a better way." Percival insisted, however, that it was time to "review our whole approach to the game, at all levels, if we are to keep pace with the ever developing hockey structure."

Not long after the 1972 series ended, Bruce Kidd and John Macfarlane published *The Death of Hockey*, the most devastating historical analysis ever written on Canadian hockey and a radical recipe for overhauling the game. The authors blamed the NHL for hijacking Canada's game and declared that the focus on profit making was threatening to irrevocably damage hockey at all levels. They backed up their thesis with a detailed analysis of the very problems that Percival had been trying to solve for years; however, Percival was referred to only as an expert coach whose voice had not been heard. The authors failed to recognize Percival's thirty year campaign to modernize the NHL, and when they stated, "(in Canada) we do not debate hockey strategy. We have no leaders in the scientific development of the game," they did a great disservice to the man who was a leader in the scientific development of hockey throughout the world.

Given Kidd and Macfarlane's oversight, it is not surprising that of the dozen books written about the 1972 Canada/Russia Series, only Roy MacSkimming's *Cold War: The Amazing Canada – Soviet Hockey Series*, and Martin Lawrence's *The Red Machine* even begin to explore Percival's role in the development of hockey in Canada and the Soviet Union. Jack Ludwig, in his book *Hockey Night in Moscow*, gives Percival a brief introduction as an overlooked Canadian fitness expert but admits that when asked by Russian editors, "who were the Tarasov's of Canada?" he was reduced to mumbling nonsense. Ludwig also discusses a tour he and Ken Dryden took of the Red Army Club in Moscow where they discovered training methods that were unheard of in Canada. Dryden is said to have told the author, "Nobody ever told him what to do to develop the muscles and bone articulations essential to top goaltending. Nobody had ever made any sense to him calisthenically speaking." Yet Ken Dryden's father, Murray, was a member of The Fitness Institute and knew Percival well; Ken's brother, Dave, had been a member and one of Percival's prized pupils for eight years, and Ken himself had gone through a battery of tests at The Fitness Institute as a member of Fr. Bauer's National Team in 1970. Why was it so difficult for anyone examining Canadian hockey, even insightful critics such as Kidd, Macfarlane and Dryden, to acknowledge what Percival was doing and had been doing for almost thirty years?

While Percival was "looked upon as some kind of witch-doctor" in Canada, Anatoly Tarasov had earned the title of "ice doctor" in the Soviet Union after absorbing everything he could find that was written by Percival and incorporating it into his Russian hockey manuals. Those Canadians who were alarmed by what they witnessed in the 1972 Summit Series bypassed Willowdale and headed straight for Moscow. Fred Shero, "the reigning intellectual" in Canadian hockey during the 1970s, was one of them. He rightfully concluded, "While the Russians and the Europeans have made a science of the game, we continue to stumble along blindly with primitive ideas that should have been discarded a long time ago." Yet, Fred Shero, who credited Percival's books and pamphlets with helping him develop his knowledge of hockey, didn't go to The Fitness Institute to talk with the Canadian who had written those books and pamphlets and who had introduced the science of hockey to the Russians and the Europeans. Shero ran off to Russia to become an acolyte of Percival's finest student, Anotoly Tarasov. Instead of re-reading *The Hockey Handbook*, Shero boasted, "I must have read

(*Tarasov's Road to Olympus*) a thousand times." Roger Nielson, who would inherit Shero's mantle in the intellectually challenged NHL, was coaching junior hockey in Peterborough at that time with the help of "old Russian hockey-training manuals." Years later, Nielson was reported to have assisted a minor hockey coach by giving him a copy of *The Hockey Handbook*. Nielson informed the man that it was a book that "Percival wrote on the Russian system."

Some of the Canadians who embarked on pilgrimages to Moscow heard the name Lloyd Percival for the very first time while attending lectures by Soviet hockey officials. A lot of time and money could have been saved if they had simply driven to Willowdale and sat down with Percival in his office – the same office where Percival and Tarasov discussed hockey training on a number of occasions and where Tarasov gave Percival a copy of his book, *Road To Olympus (1969)*, with an inscription that began:

> Respectively to Lloyd:
>
> Your wonderful book which introduced us to the mysteries of Canadian Hockey, I have read like a schoolboy. Thank you for a hockey science which is significant to hockey world.

The following year Tarasov took time out from a tour with the Russian team and spent fourteen hours with Percival at The Fitness Institute. At this meeting, Percival expressed mock displeasure that his hockey handbook was so widely used in the Soviet Union and translations were sold but he received no financial compensation, while Tarasov was in North America promoting a book based on Percival's ideas in order to increase the royalties he would take back to Russia. Tarasov is said to have replied, "Lloyd you live under the wrong system."

A Return Engagement in Detroit

It is not surprising that people assumed that Percival's return to the NHL in the fall of 1972 was a result of the publicity regarding his influence on Soviet hockey. The truth was that Detroit had finalized arrangements with Percival prior to the end of the previous NHL season, and he had met with the Red Wing players and laid out his program before Team Canada was even selected. "All Russia did was to point up that we were on the right road," a Detroit executive told the *Globe and Mail*.

Management from top to bottom said they were committed to the project. Owner Bruce Norris, son of "Big" Jim Norris, had witnessed the work Percival had done with the team in the glory years of the 1950s. The Vice President in Charge of Operations for the Detroit Red Wings was former "Sports College" employee, Jim Bishop, whom Norris had first hired to operate his lacrosse franchise before moving him over to the hockey team. Bishop credited Percival with teaching him that "there is no value in a dogmatic attachment to the old ways," and the hiring of Ned Harkness, coach of the NCAA champion Cornell University hockey team, definitely raised eyebrows around the NHL. Harkness was also an NCAA champion coach in lacrosse and the only coach in the history of the NCAA with national championships in two sports.

In 1970, Harkness was named head coach of the Detroit Red Wings and asked to infuse "sophistication" into NHL coaching. In many ways, he was a breath of fresh air in the stale ranks of NHL coaches. Unfortunately, as with Bishop, his experience was with younger athletes and in a time when changing attitudes towards personal grooming and dress codes were making life difficult for many coaches, Harkness and Bishop proved to be particularly rigid and ill-prepared to deal with adult NHL hockey players. Before he had completed his first season behind the bench, Harkness was kicked upstairs and replaced by Doug Barkley. Harkness then fired Barkley and replaced him with former Red Wing player, Johnny Wilson, before the end of the 1971-1972 season. Wilson was a devotee of "Sports College" and was thrilled to learn that Bruce Norris had given Percival a two-year mandate to develop and oversee the training of the Red Wings, along with all of the teams in the Detroit farm system, and had authorized Percival to spend $150,000 on a training facility for the Detroit Olympia where the Red Wings practiced and played.

With seeming stability under Bishop, Harkness and Wilson, Percival presented his program to the Detroit players in the spring of 1971-1972, reporting that they "responded as I knew they would – with enthusiasm, including the older players." He later admitted that the summer training program presented to the players was a complete departure from anything they had ever been asked to do and proved to be a tough sell. It was always Percival's expressed belief that NHL players were smart enough, and dedicated enough, to take on whatever was in their best interests, and he repeatedly blamed coaches and management for the failure of his programs. In Detroit, his convictions were shared by his former lieutenant, Jim Bishop, who also believed that management was behind the times and that athletes had become more open minded and ready to accept new ideas. The reality was that neither NHL management, nor NHL players as a group, were comfortable with radical changes in the way hockey players trained.

Percival's goal with the Red Wings was to create "an effort and performance tempo never achieved in hockey, of any classification" and to prepare the team "to be able to play four periods, instead of just three." In training camp, Wilson worked the players harder than they were used to, but said that they didn't mind because they weren't bored by the monotony of typical NHL practices. The Red Wings won the first four games of the season, outscoring the opposition twenty-two to eight. A lot of the credit was given to Coach Wilson, who was not afraid to share the credit with Percival, whom he said "knew as much about physical fitness as any authority in the world." Harkness was also free with his praise for Percival. When a sportswriter asked him if he (Harkness) had taken "a few pages out of the Soviet Union's hockey book," he responded:

> Hell no. But like the Russians, we have made use of Lloyd Percival's knowledge on physical fitness.
>
> For years people in the National Hockey League treated Percival like he was the quack doctor in a medicine show, not one of the world's foremost authorities on fitness.

By Christmas, the rest of the teams in the NHL had played themselves into better shape, and it became clear that the Red Wings, who were not a very talented group of players, would be hard-pressed to make the playoffs. Bishop had told Percival from the beginning that he was not looking for instant success, and Percival believed that everyone understood that this was a long-term project. That didn't stop the fans and the media in Detroit from making life miserable for Harkness and Bishop, neither of who had any experience with this kind of pressure. They, in turn, put pressure on Wilson and everyone began to lose sight of the long-term plan, although Wilson insisted that he stuck with Percival's program, and that it was working. He later said that he was amazed that, "with the talent on the team, we were in contention at all."

The breaking point came after Wilson honoured a promise to give the players some much needed rest if they won an important game. This was an aspect of Percival's philosophy that Wilson believed was particularly relevant to the long grind of an NHL schedule. Bishop and Harkness, on the other hand, were evangelists for Percival's ideas regarding intensity and scientific training but never really bought into his theories about the need for proper mental and physical recovery. They were furious. Within days, Wilson had become the fourth straight Detroit coach to be fired before the end of the season, and Percival was nowhere to be found.

Ironically, it was Wilson who became the villain of record. In the February 1974 edition of *SFI*, Percival announced that he wanted to "set the record straight" about his time in Detroit in light of "disturbing and inaccurate statements" that were "creating an impression that the training methods used were not compatible with the needs of an NHL hockey club." Percival wrote that it was Wilson's ego that led to the abandonment of the program, and it became widely accepted that Wilson had given his bosses an ultimatum: "either Percival goes, or I go." Wilson denied issuing the ultimatum, did not recall that that there were any problems between him and Percival and insisted that he carried on with Percival's program until the day he was fired. As much as he probably upset Percival by introducing his own ideas to Percival's program, Wilson was the only coach in the league capable of understanding and implementing the program as a holistic unit. Percival would have come to terms with Wilson's modifications – after all, Wilson was the coach – and any problems between the two could have been ironed out with the help of Bishop and Harkness. In spite of their supposed loyalty to Percival, it would seem that they were responsible for exacerbating the situation – if not actually creating it – and set Wilson up to be the fall guy. What was supposed to be a two-year program aimed at helping the Red Wings regain their status as an NHL powerhouse became a casualty of front office machinations and further justification for the NHL to proclaim that Percival's methods would not work with Canadian professional hockey players.

Special Delivery and Rhythmics

D URING ONE OF HIS STOPOVERS in Detroit in 1972, Percival stepped into the hotel bar and heard a soft rock group called Special Delivery. The band and especially the lead singer, Connie Graham, impressed him so much that he invited them to Toronto and offered to manage and promote them north of the border. By the spring of 1973, Percival had pulled together a group of financial backers which included Al Balding and Jim Gairdner. Special Delivery began appearing in clubs and hotel lounges around Toronto and was booked for a week in Halifax. At one of the Toronto dates, Percival assembled a group of reporters and veterans of the entertainment business. He regaled them with stories about his own time playing banjo and dancing on stage at the end of the 1920s and explained that managing the group was like coaching, that it was helping to fill the void left from giving up track and field coaching in 1967. Percival also used the occasion to announce his plans for Special Delivery to raise money for the Olympic Trust.

By the fall, Special Delivery was at the centre of another new fitness promotion: Rhythmics. Percival dressed the group in Roman costumes, called them Olympus and co-wrote with them two six minute songs, "Stop It Draggin' " and "Hippocrates," recorded on alternate sides of a 45 rpm record. The record, professionally packaged in a 9×12 heavy gauge folder which also included a number of colourful 8 1/2 by 11 inch pages devoted to specific exercises, was the centrepiece of a Rhythmics fitness package that Percival explained would "solve the greatest of all fitness problems – finding an effective home program you can stay with." Percival announced that Rhythmics was an "entirely new concept," in which the combination of "dance/exercise movements" was integrated "with original music and lyrics designed to combine the physical and mental benefits of exercise with the motivational effect of music." He planned to market the package to schools, community centres and daycare centres, as well as to individuals in their homes. In January 1974, 5,000 people reportedly attended a presentation at Sherway Gardens in Mississauga where Olympus performed the music while Val and Sandra Bezic demonstrated the fitness routines. The Bezics told reporters at the time that the fitness routine was very effective and a lot of fun. Today, however, Val recalls that the routine was great but the music was "hokey." He remembers being mildly embarrassed and feels that Percival could have used help from music professionals. Although the concept was innovative and prescient, a precursor to the "aerobics craze" and the Jane Fonda videos of the 1980s, Rhythmics had little chance of catching on. The presentation, including Roman costumes and lyrics with references to classical Greece, was not really in tune with the times, and even Percival's closest associates questioned the wisdom of the project. In fact, not one other project in his career was greeted with more skepticism than was his association with Special Delivery and Rhythmics.

A Fitness Institute Without Lloyd Percival

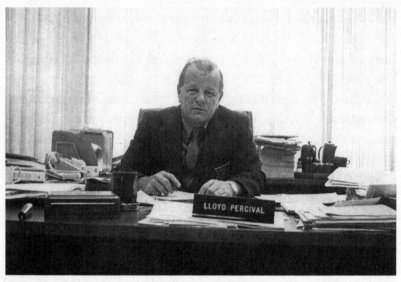

Lloyd Percival at his desk in the corner office at the
Willowdale Fitness Institute, c. 1972.

P ERCIVAL HAD ALWAYS SEEMED TO BE ABLE to squeeze more work out
of a day than the rest of us. His ability to inspire those around
him to work tirelessly on his behalf and his ability to juggle
numerous projects at the same time contributed to the remarkable
range of his accomplishments. This meant that he was constantly up
against deadlines and placed a tremendous amount of stress on the
people who worked with him. Wink McRoberts was Percival's secretary when he worked out of the house on Glen Road, and again at
The Fitness Institute in Willowdale. She recalls a man who thrived
under the pressure and did his best work when he left things to the

last minute. Alyce Tweedley also provided secretarial services for Percival along with her future husband, Doug MacLennan. She too recalled how the charismatic Percival could inspire those around him to devote whatever time and effort was required to complete his many projects. Unfortunately, Percival was not nearly as effective when delegating. Generally, he assigned tasks, not projects. Even Joe Taylor and Doug MacLennan, who did so much of the work required to complete Percival's projects, were all too often forced to wait for their boss to provide his input and add the finishing touches.

When Percival began work on the *sports & fitness Instructor* in 1972, he was deeply involved with the Detroit Red Wings. He was consulting to an ever expanding list of individual athletes, sports organizations and groups. He had a list of seven proposed book titles on his desk. He was working with the COA on Game Plan and actively seeking corporate sponsorship for the large scale, national fitness program on which he had been working. He was running the most advanced health and fitness club in the world with a second Fitness Institute in Mississauga in the planning stages, and he continued to entertain the media whenever they came calling. Something had to give. When Percival morphed into a music pro-moter a few months later, it did.

When the Willowdale facility first opened, Percival had chosen the corner office on the main floor because he said it offered him a view of everyone who came and went and allowed the members to see the face of The Fitness Institute. Whether he would have admit-ted to it or not, when Percival moved his office upstairs to Fitness Institute Productions early in 1972, it signalled that he was losing interest in the more mundane activities of The Fitness Institute. The majority of the staff and members failed to notice any appre-ciable change in the way the Institute operated, and to say that it was anything less than the "Temple of Fitness" it had been when it first opened would be doing a disservice to Percival, Jim Gairdner, Doug MacLennan and the staff. But The Fitness Institute was too complex an entity to maintain such high standards without full-time direction from the top, and Percival was not the only guiding figure whose absence was becoming conspicuous.

At the same time that Percival was becoming less and less involved in day-to-day operations, Jim Gairdner had tired of the corporate world and sought the serenity and self-sufficiency of his working farm and woodworking shop in Cheltenham. Without Jim Gairdner, there would never have been a Fitness Institute, not at the Inn on the Park, not in Willowdale and not in Mississauga. Percival told Charles Taylor in 1973, "I don't think I would have made it if it hadn't been for Jim Gairdner – not just his money but his practical advice and his whole approach." Gairdner shared Percival's faith that what they were building was important to Canadian society because the success of its athletes and the health and welfare of its citizens were essential to the future of the country, and it was a rare day that Percival and Gairdner did not sit down together, at least for a brief chat. The chats ended when Percival moved upstairs, and Gairdner moved to the farm.

Jim Gairdner asked his son, Bill, to move into The Fitness Institute and supervise the financial and contractual operations. Bill Gairdner's time with the Don Mills Track Club had made him a devoted follower of Percival. After he moved on to university in the United States, Gairdner abided by the training program Percival had devised for him, still remembers Percival as a kind of surrogate father and, to this day, practices many of the things he learned from Percival. By 1973, however, Bill Gairdner was comfortably ensconced in a world far removed from sports and business. After earning a PhD in Comparative Literature from Stanford University, he had accepted a tenure stream appointment at York University. When his father asked him to take his place at The Fitness Institute, Bill's first instinct was to say no. His sense of filial duty caused him to change his mind.

There is a myth attached to The Fitness Institute that Jim Gairdner was the strong financial figure that kept Percival in check. Bill Gairdner admits that although his father was successful in the brokerage business, he was a dreamer and a philanthropist, better at giving money away than counting it. He had a reputation within the family for "letting money flow through his fingers like sand." When Bill Gairdner moved into The Fitness Institute in the spring of 1973, he felt like he had arrived at the beach. All of the services were first class, but no one was counting the money that came in and went out. Jim Gairdner's long-time business advisor and Fitness Institute Treasurer, Aubrey Montgomery, was still prowling the corridors annoying people with petty concerns over wastage; however, unbeknownst to the staff, Montgomery was an engineer not an accountant, had no idea of the big picture and had led the elder Gairdner into making some questionable financial decisions.

Bill Gairdner brought in a financial analyst to examine the books while he became acquainted with the staff and the operations. He saw fantastic state-of-the-art equipment that was under-utilized, unparalleled customer care that was not paying for itself, golf members who treated The Fitness Institute like a private gentleman's club, a record system that was bloated and ineffective, a publishing division that employed twelve people but produced only one monthly publication, and he saw empty lockers. Bill Gairdner realized that changes would have to be made, and the staff sensed it. The staff was loyal to Percival, but some were more loyal than others. Everyone wondered about Bill Gairdner's qualifications for the job, and some were convinced that he was determined to "take over" and make it his Fitness Institute. While it is true that Bill was more interested in linking the Gairdner name with The Fitness Institute than his father had ever been and referred to it as "my father's business," it is not fair to say that he was intent on diminishing Percival's contribution. He had too much respect for his former coach.

The younger Gairdner decided that he couldn't wait for the financial reports before making changes. Cutting staff was certainly part of it, but so too was adding staff. Sales staff is an integral aspect of any fitness club today, but The Fitness Institute had always relied on Percival's reputation and the considerable publicity he generated to attract members. While this had been enough to fill the Inn on the Park, the Willowdale location was bigger and more isolated. Bill Gairdner hired sales people, initially from the Gairdner brokerage firm, before realizing that sales people who were more in tune with the fitness business were better suited. One of the very first to be hired was Bill Salter, who stayed on for twenty-four years. Salter's background was in the investment business, but he was also a competitive athlete; he saw the business from the member viewpoint as well as from the management perspective and shared with Bill Gairdner a perception that things were top heavy and inefficient. According to Salter, Percival "kept throwing people at it (The Fitness Institute) and hoped that it would manage itself."

When the financial reports arrived, the outlook proved to be worse than was expected. The analysis concluded that The Fitness Institute in Willowdale, together with the yet to be opened Mississauga facility, could bankrupt the Gairdner family within a decade if major changes were not made. It wasn't simply a problem of balancing income with expenses in Willowdale, the utilization of space on the second floor of the building was an issue, and more significantly, the family faced a huge financial crisis due to bad leasing deals at both the Willowdale and Mississauga locations. Drastic changes in these financial arrangements had to be made for there to be any chance of The Fitness Institute becoming financially viable.

Percival had nothing to do with the leases; he was never supposed to be involved in the financial management, nor in selling memberships, and everyone knew that he was not cut out to be a manager. Bill Gairdner knew that these things bored Percival and were a waste of his talents but was also aware that Percival never tired of spending money. It was not that Percival was unreasonable in his demands. It was just that his vision and his ego always demanded the best. When he started spending much of his time as well as The Fitness Institute's money on Special Delivery and Rhythmics, even his closest friends and most loyal supporters recognized a problem and wondered if he was going through a delayed mid-life crisis. Bill

Gairdner "thought that Lloyd had lost his moral bearings – he just wasn't there – he had already absented himself."

Jim Gairdner wasn't there either. When Bill would call to explain the problems to him, his father would reply that he couldn't deal with it; he was too busy "bringing in the hay." It took almost a year, but Bill Gairdner came to the painful decision that the best thing would be for Percival to be bought out. He felt like a "patricide" but was convinced that it was necessary for the future of his family. After explaining this to his father, Bill managed to get Jim and Lloyd into Jim's office for a meeting. Jim Gairdner explained the situation to Lloyd and offered to buy him out. Bill remembers the figure as $100,000, and that it wasn't really a buyout because the financial status of the company rendered Percival's shares worthless. The money came from Jim Gairdner's personal account and was more of a "payoff" for all that Percival had done for The Fitness Institute. Percival was also left with ownership of FI Productions and the offices upstairs. According to Bill Gairdner, Percival accepted immediately.

Lloyd's daughter, Jan, has always maintained that her father was badly mistreated, that the value of The Fitness Institute was understated and the payoff inadequate. There is no question that the unique nature of the assets and the services of The Fitness Institute made it a valuable institution and that Percival's contribution to its position in the world of sport and fitness was worth considerably more than $100,000. It is also true that, from a business standpoint, the assessment of a bleak financial picture handed to Bill Gairdner rendered shares relatively worthless and the payoff fair.

Percival's friends believed that he accepted the financial settlement because he was worried about his health and wanted to ensure that Dorothy and Jan were financially secure. This is the story Percival told, and there is a great deal of circumstantial evidence to support it. There was the Percival legacy. He had already lived longer than his father and his older brother, both of whom died due to heart failure before either reached the age of sixty, and MacLennan remembers an incident towards the end when they "were walking down the hall at The Fitness Institute and Lloyd suddenly put his hand out on the wall – caught himself – and then continued on. 'I think I've just had a TIA (a mini-stroke),' Percival said." Joe Taylor also recalls Percival's concern over his heart and the family history, the heart medication and the oxygen inhaler in his office.

The public knew nothing about Percival's health concerns and little about changes at The Fitness Institute. Even though he was no longer officially attached to The Fitness Institute, Percival's star continued to rise, and he worked at a frenetic pace. When a small group of prominent Canadians was polled for their opinions on the upcoming federal election, Percival was amongst them. And when Al Gilbert, Canada's professional photographer of the year for 1974, assembled his portfolio of twenty-six photographs "most representative of Canadians today," Lloyd Percival was amongst them. Along with all of his ongoing projects, Percival was reported to be working with World Hockey Association (WHA) President, Gary Davidson, and the league's marquee player, Bobby Hull, on a development program to be implemented by every team in the league with the first phase, a program for the players preparing for the WHA's version of a Canada/Russia summit series set for September 1974. He was also busy with preparations for a meeting with representatives of a major corporation in Montreal on July 13 to discuss his national fitness program. This was to be "a mammoth nationwide fitness project that would include television shows, books, booklets, records and cassettes, traveling clinics and other projects," according to Joe Taylor. The Percival family expected it to be a "million dollar project" and the new central focus for Lloyd.

Previously, Doug MacLennan would have accompanied Percival on the trip to Montreal, but MacLennan was still an employee of The Fitness Institute and no longer Percival's right-hand man. On the evening of July 12, Percival asked Bob Bursach to accompany him on the five hour train ride. Bursach was also busy with Fitness Institute business. It was one of the few times in his life that it happened, but Percival travelled to Montreal alone.

Goodbye Dear Coach

N O MATTER WHAT ANYONE RECALLED regarding Percival's health, no one was prepared for the terrible shock when Jim Gairdner made an unscheduled appearance at The Fitness Institute on the afternoon of July 13, 1974, called the department heads into his office and informed them that Lloyd Percival had collapsed while attending a business luncheon in Montreal. He had been rushed to the Royal Victoria Hospital and pronounced dead at 3:40 in the afternoon. Although there was some confusion at first as to whether he had choked or suffered a heart attack, the coroner concluded that Lloyd Percival died of heart failure.

To the general public who only knew Percival through the media, there was a different kind of shock, just as there was when Jim Fixx, the father of the jogging craze in the United States, died of a heart attack while jogging. People do not expect a fitness guru to die of a heart attack at the age of sixty-one. Unfortunately, Percival's death, like Fixx's death, allowed some to discount the teachings and discouraged others from promoting the legacy. In addition, the image of Percival as a chain smoker was so powerful that some saw him as an architect of his own demise and likewise discounted his authority – there are people today, some of whom were close to Percival, who still believe that he died of lung cancer.

Percival's sudden death was a national story and front page news in Montreal and Toronto. There were long obituaries that presented some of the highlights of his eventful career and discussed his outspokenness and lack of recognition in Canada; there was also a heartfelt sense of personal loss from the numerous columnists and sportswriters who had come to know him well. Jim Proudfoot's banner read, "Lloyd Percival was a genius we overlooked." While extolling Percival's virtues, Proudfoot did not shy away from revealing what he saw as Percival's "Achilles heel":

> Percival refused to soften his bluntness. And he believed his flair for publicity was an asset. Faced with a hassle, he never took the diplomatic way out. He couldn't stop competing.

Douglas Fisher lamented the loss of "one of the half dozen greatest Canadians of the past thirty years" and echoed Proudfoot's assessment of Percival's tragic flaw:

> He was difficult because he was absolute. He lacked the one pervasive, peculiarly Canadian talent. He didn't compromise easily.

Although he included the least facts, Dick Beddoes came the closest to capturing the man and penned the most poignant tribute with a flourish that Percival would have loved and only Beddoes could pull off:

> The beginning of no Canadian Open golf tournament should be allowed to deflect us from the task at hand.

> Canadian Opens are born every year, but a Lloyd Percival dies only once. It is part of the courtesy to tip the typewriter goodbye.

> Super salesman, coach, irritant, self-promoter, innovator, physical-jerk philosopher – these were a few of the designations cut to fit the squat dean of the old "Sports College" of Canada.

> Percival belonged, in sum to that tiny band of evangelists, the John Browns, the Aimee Semple McPhersons, the Conn Smythes – who have extra-human wellsprings of force. As a rule their

temporal stay is tempestuous. They feel obliged, as the early Samuel Butler suggested to: "… prove their doctrine orthodox. By apostolic blows and knocks …

Besides his family, it was the athletes and The Fitness Institute staff who were affected most personally by Percival's sudden death, and Roberta Picco (Angeloni) spoke for them in the final edition of the *sports & fitness Instructor* (September 1974), half of which was devoted to a tribute to its founder. Titled, "We called him 'Coach,'" Picco's eulogy touched on Percival's public career, but it was her personal reflections that were most revealing:

> You were my coach. You were my boss. But to me you were also my friend. I shared some of the greatest moments of my life with you; you also pulled me through many defeats. When I became disillusioned with sport, you motivated me into trying again.
>
> You taught me many things about myself and about people. You encouraged me to compete and to strive, because that is what you did. You taught me not to fear failure, or success. Failure, you said, is part of winning if you learn from your mistakes. Everyone has hurdles to overcome, you said, but only those who do become winners. And you were a winner. … You were a beautiful human being. My heart is filled with sorrow for you – but I'm happy just to have known you.
>
> Goodbye dear Coach.

As with his mentor, Knute Rockne, who was eulogized as "an artist as well as a football coach," the outpouring of grief following Percival's death extended well beyond the sporting community. The most moving and in many ways, the most insightful tributes were written by *Toronto Sun* Entertainment Editor, George Anthony, and *Sun* columnist, Joan Sutton.

Sutton focused on her first memories of Lloyd and Dorothy with the Red Devils in the early 1950s. She recalled the first time that she met Lloyd:

> When I think of Lloyd, I think of him with his wife, Do, and I see them, surrounded by young people. That was how they were the night that I met them, and I have never been in their home when it wasn't like that. They offered warmth, understanding and, for many, a foothold on life.

Sutton's column attempted to reveal the aspects of Percival that were not often found in the sports columns: "that he was a man – a warm, loveable, funny, demanding, loyal and giving man." It was this side of Percival that Sutton remembered most, the side of him which was not devoted to creating world champions and gold medal winners but to developing better human beings. Sutton explained, if you wanted to know "more, perhaps, than you'll discover about him in any list of achievements, disappointments, or controversies," you just had to listen to the words of his favourite song, "Sweet Georgia Brown":

> No gal made has got a shade
> on sweet Georgia Brown
> Two left feet, but oh so neat,
> That's sweet Georgia Brown...

Toronto nightclub performer, Ruby Ramsey Ross, played an "almost Dixieland version" of "Sweet Georgia Brown" at Percival's funeral. She also played "Rambling Rose," "When the Saints Go Marching In" and "Cruising Down the River." George Anthony wrote about the funeral and described how the unusual proceedings befitted such an unusual man. He wrote about Percival's work with Special Delivery and quoted Percival on how working with the young musicians allowed him to combine his passion for music with his love of coaching young people. Anthony wanted his readers to understand why when people referred to Percival as "Coach," the term carried so much resonance, "not just to his Olympic athletes but to all of (those) whom he trained in his special way." Anthony learned about Percival's death from jazz pianist Billy Stephenson and wrote, "I think Lloyd would have dug that too, that I got the word not from a newscast, not from a sports writer, but from a young musician."

As in life, where Percival's addiction to publicity was in direct contrast to his lack of interest in the traditional trappings of success, the ragtime funeral surprised most people. In deference to wishes he had shared with Dorothy numerous times over the years, the celebration of Percival's life was followed by internment in an unmarked grave at Toronto's Mount Pleasant Cemetery.

PART IV

Legacy

When Canada was at Last Ready for Him

JIM PROUDFOOT LAMENTED that Lloyd Percival's death came "just when all his old adversaries were ready for defeat (and) when Canada was at last ready for him." Percival has continued to shape Canadian physical culture and the role it plays in the larger cultural mosaic, and his fingerprints can still be found on major developments in amateur and professional sport forty years after his death. However, his name is rarely spoken and historians treat him as a footnote, dusted off only in times of controversy, such as the Ben Johnson scandal and the inquiry into the use of steroids in track and field in 1988. Proudfoot's eulogy provided one explanation as to why acceptance for Percival and his ideas came so late in his life and why that acceptance remains less than complete:

> (Percival) never lacked enemies. Or, to put it
> another way, he was his own worst enemy. He
> never learned a basic fact that nobody likes to hear
> an unpleasant truth. ...

> There's no question his abrasive personality cost
> him the acceptance he needed to get his ideas
> across. People were so busy raging at him, or
> questioning his motives, they didn't hear what he
> was saying.

Canadians do not like people who are too loud, too confident and too often correct. We don't like listening to them, we don't like following their advice, and we certainly don't like acknowledging our debt to them. And there is much for which Canadians are indebted to Lloyd Percival.

The Business of Fitness and the Health of a Nation

IT WAS FORTUNATE FOR THE FITNESS INSTITUTE that Bill Gairdner had been at his desk for more than year and had already begun to institute changes when Percival died. Given that the overall financial picture was so bleak, the magnificent institution that Percival and Jim Gairdner built may never have recovered. Within days of his father breaking the news to the department heads and word spreading amongst the staff, Bill Gairdner held a meeting of the entire staff at the nearby Ramada Inn. He explained the precarious financial position of The Fitness Institute, the need to streamline operations and the difficult decision to cut staff by fifty percent.

Rick Johnson, who had been studying with Dr. Shephard at the University of Toronto when Percival hired him in 1969, was at that meeting. Like Dave Steen, another former Don Mills athlete who had joined The Fitness Institute staff, and Bill Salter, Johnson gives a great deal of credit for the survival of The Fitness Institute to the leadership provided by Bill Gairdner (Johnson, Steen and Salter were key figures in the post-Percival era of The Fitness Institute). Even Doug MacLennan, who never regained the status and respect he had received while working side-by-side with Percival, recognized the need for these changes and was content that the demands of the service model he and Percival had established in 1963 were not compromised by the new financial model introduced by Bill Gairdner.

One of the most difficult situations facing Gairdner was how to deal with Jan Percival. Jan shared something with Bill Gairdner. She was the "boss's daughter." Jan hadn't suddenly appeared in the executive suite, however. She had worked her way up the ladder to the position of Director of Women's Programs and was well-respected by the staff and membership. When Bill Gairdner arrived on the scene, she naturally bristled. Just as Bill was out to protect his father's interests, Jan was intent on protecting Coach's stake. It would have taken a great deal of dialogue and conciliation for them to work together, and it seems that neither was interested. After Lloyd died, the situation became untenable, and Jan was soon out the door. She still feels that her departure was manipulated and that, like her father, she was poorly compensated for her years of service.

No matter how firmly Bill Gairdner put his stamp, as well as his family name, on The Fitness Institute and contributed to its survival after Percival's death, it still was, and would remain for a very long time, "Lloyd Percival's Fitness Institute." The members knew it, and the elite athletes who trained there after his death knew it. The fact that Dave Podborski, Jocelyn Lovell and so many other athletes who trained at The Fitness Institute were winning national and international competitions throughout the latter half of the 1970s and into the 1980s is another legacy of Lloyd Percival. The technical backing, combined with the supportive environment that Roger Jackson talked about at the Inn on the Park and so many athletes remember in Willowdale, was crucial to the development of elite athletes in Canada. No other such environment existed in Canada until Calgary inherited the Olympic Oval and Sports Complex as a legacy of the 1984 Winter Olympics. Also In 1984, Bill Gairdner fulfilled one of the long-time dreams of his father and Lloyd Percival when The Fitness Institute was named Canada's first, "national testing centre for Canadian high-performance athletes."

Let us not forget either that the concept of a "fitness institute" rather than a "health club" which Percival and Jim Gairdner introduced to the world in 1963 completely reshaped the way we think about personal fitness, spawned a vast array of imitators and helped give birth to the vast fitness industry we have today.

The Fitness Institute spearheaded the drive to make fitness an integral part of corporate culture in Canada. This is an area where Bill Gairdner and John Wildman made tremendous progress after Percival died; however, Percival first introduced the concept of selling "Personnel Fitness" programs to the business world through "Sports College" in 1951, and the Inn on the Park had a limited corporate fitness program. The first company to fully embrace the concept and to subsidize fitness club memberships for its employees was Murray Koffler's, Koffler's Stores Ltd. When the new Fitness Institute opened in Willowdale in 1969, Koffler moved his head office into the building because he believed "corporations are more likely to flourish when those who direct it are in good shape and health." Major corporations, including Shell Canada and General Foods, had also become clients of The Fitness Institute prior to Percival's death.

Koffler's partner at the Inn on the Park, Isadore Sharpe, was recently cited by Roger Martin, former Dean of the Rotman School of Management at the University of Toronto, as one of the best examples of businessmen who have dramatically improved upon prevailing business models by employing "integrative thinking." Sharpe is now in his eighties but could pass for a man of sixty. He remains the CEO of the Four Seasons chain of hotels and is living life to the fullest. Sharpe could be a poster boy for what he calls "the Lloyd Percival school for understanding your body." Percival taught Sharpe that fitness for him was about "finding a comfortable level" and understanding "the mind-body connection." Sharpe believes that this has led to a lifetime of better health, better business, better sex and a better attitude to living every day. Sharpe also believes that the tremendous success enjoyed by Four Season's Hotels has something to do with the fitness sessions and philosophical discussions he engaged in with Lloyd Percival in the 1960s.

The health and fitness of millions of Canadians who never met Percival but who listened to him on the radio, watched him on television or read his articles in the newspaper, and the generations that have followed is also part of Percival's legacy. The fact that we have sixty, seventy and even eighty year olds competing in marathons and triathlons, or even just going to the gym three times a week, can be traced back to the 1950s when Percival began his campaign to convince Canadians that thirty-five was not middle-aged and that out-of-shape thirty and forty year olds could become fit, healthy individuals; that fitness did not have to be about sport and competition, it could simply be a means of getting the most out of life. Percival also stripped away myths regarding femininity, fitness and sport. He led the way in unfettering Canadian society from pervasive attitudes regarding gender, middle age and physical activity. And even he might be surprised at how successful this campaign has been.

The 1976 Montreal Olympics

A s Percival had predicted, preparations for the 1976 Olympics proved to be too little and too late. Canada earned the dubious distinction of being the first host country not to win a gold medal. Whether the changes Percival would have preferred to see in Game Plan could have made a difference is debatable. The Canadian team finished in eleventh place in the official points ranking and the eleven medals won by Canadians – five silver and six bronze – was the highest total since 1932.

Swimmers won eight of the eleven Canadian medals because as Percival had stated in 1952, the Canadian Swimming Association (CSA) was one of only two sports federations in Canada "strong enough to work independently of the COA." When all of the government policy initiatives were put forward after 1968, the CSA governing body was already well-organized and able to take full advantage of new funding opportunities. As Roger Jackson told the *Globe and Mail* in August 1973, "swimming is a bit different because it's organized better than any other amateur sport in Canada."

Canada's other medals in Montreal were a bronze won by Michel Vaillancourt in equestrian dressage, the famous silver medal won by high jumper Greg Joy and the less famous silver medal won by canoeist John Wood in the 500 Metre C1. Wood was one of more than a dozen Canadian athletes competing in Montreal who had regularly passed through the doors of Percival's Fitness Institute in the years leading up to the Olympics. His medal came as a surprise to most Canadians, but there were some very good reasons for Wood's performance and one of them was Lloyd Percival.

Canoeing was the other sport Percival had praised in 1952 for its independence of the COA. Ken Lane and Bert Oldershaw, both of whom had trained under Percival prior to the 1952 Olympics, became important figures in the administration of the sport after their competitive days were over. When Jim Mossman was asked to coach the 1960 Olympic Team, he accepted the position on condition that he could use Percival as a consultant. In an era when Canadian amateur sports bodies had no ongoing national coach positions and simply named an honorary coach on the eve of each international competition, Mossman was a rarity. He was the Olympic coach in 1960, 1964 and 1968, coached the 1972 Olympic Team during the months preceding the Games and accompanied the team to Munich, attended the Montreal Olympics in 1976 in his capacity as Technical Director of the CCA and led Canadian teams at numerous other international competitions.

Throughout these years, Mossman was in constant contact with Percival and frequently brought paddlers to The Fitness Institute for testing and training programs. Through him, as well as through the voices of Lane and Oldershaw, Percival exerted a profound influence on the development of flat water canoe racing in Canada. In spite of the up-to-date coaching methods that Percival helped Mossman bring to the training of paddlers in Canada, Canadian competitors had difficulty gaining a spot in the finals of international competitions during the 1960s. The sheer volume of paddlers in Eastern Europe (there were 50,000 registered in Hungary alone compared to 4,000 in Canada), the year-round training, the advanced work of the sport scientists, which by the 1970s included the extensive use of ergogenic aids, and the regular competition facilitated by the ideological compatibility and physical proximity of the countries left Canada at a distinct disadvantage. Still, as was the case with the swimming federation, the CCA was sufficiently evolved in 1968 to respond quickly and effectively to the new funding opportunities announced in Ottawa. They invested in a permanent winter training camp in Florida and sent their best prospects to train and compete in Europe throughout the summers.

John Wood was one of the paddlers who wintered in Florida and summered in Europe. He also visited The Fitness Institute many times and recalls that Percival was "very influential in our training." Wood credited Percival with helping him and his coach, Mac Hickox, understand "the whole concept of systematic training." On one of his visits, Percival filmed Wood paddling in the swimming pool and used a breakdown of the film to teach Wood that the sport was "more about strength than power" and to identify which muscles required specific development. John Wood won the silver medal in Montreal through his own talent and determination as well as the excellent work of coaches from Jim Mossman to Mac Hickox, but it was the foresight of the CCA and the legacy of Lloyd Percival that provided him with the opportunity.

Government Policy

PERCIVAL'S IMPACT ON GOVERNMENT POLICY in the modern era of Canadian sport has been both deep-seated and wide ranging because it was both philosophical in the promotion of sport as culture and technical in the way science has become the backbone of athletic training. Percival was a teacher and mentor to many of Canada's most influential sport bureaucrats including John Hudson, who says that "I wouldn't have gone on my scholarship without him and I wouldn't have gone on to do what I did with it." Hudson was one of the new generation of coaches, administrators and sports scientists who charted Canada's course in the modern world of amateur sport. Another was Roger Jackson who learned so much from just being around Percival in 1963 and 1964. While completing his doctoral studies at the University of Wisconsin Jackson gave credit to Percival:

> No other person in the academic or athletic
> segments of my life has been as successful, directly
> or indirectly in assisting me in my private goals.
> … My opinion of his capabilities as a coach and
> trainer, and as a "physical fitness expert" increases
> as my own knowledge expands.

Own the Podium Program: 2010, which was headed up by Roger Jackson and which engineered Canada's first truly successful Olympic experience in Vancouver, was the legacy of the pioneering work done by the new breed of sports bureaucrats who came to Ottawa in the wake of the *Task Force Report*. Dan Pugilese says that "what we are doing today is a measure of what was established back then" and "he (Percival) sparked everything that happened in Ottawa." Pugilese calls Percival "an architect," and John Hudson is convinced that Percival's "influence was far greater than anyone will ever give him credit for."

It is also in the area of government sport policy where we clearly see that Lloyd Percival was "the genius we overlooked." In spite of the tremendous impact he had on the introduction and evolution of sport policy in Canada, it was more than thirty years before people began implementing his policies, and it has taken another forty years for Canada to adopt a national sport policy that resembles the one he began espousing in 1936. *Own the Podium Program: 2010* was the first fully integrated sport development plan to be implemented in Canada, and all of the basic components are found in the proposals Percival began submitting in 1949. One of the most publicized aspects of Own the Podium was the daring assertion that Canada would rank first amongst competing nations in terms of medals won. When Canadians struggled in the early days of the Games, Jackson, who had rejected Percival's suggestion that Canada's medal aspirations be announced prior to the Montreal Olympics, was forced to defend his committee's decision on many fronts. Canadian athletes did end up winning more gold medals than any other nation – more than any in the history of the Winter Olympics – and *Own the Podium* was deemed a success.

We are still struggling to elevate Canadian summer Olympians the way we have our winter competitors, but the Road to Excellence Program has proven to be a good start, and there is reason to be optimistic after the showing of so many young Canadian competitors in London in 2012. Just think where Canadian amateur athletics would be, however, if government and sports officials had listened to Percival when he spoke out in 1936, 1944, 1949, 1952, 1958, 1964 or in 1970. There is every reason to believe that the Canadian system would be the envy of the world, and Canadian amateur athletes would bring glory to Canada on a regular basis in the 21st century.

International Hockey and "The New NHL"

T IS IN REGARD TO HOCKEY[1] that Percival's legacy is most misunderstood. While he impacted the game in ways that have never been fully appreciated, *The Hockey Handbook*, as well as everything else Percival wrote on the game, was treated with disdain by most professional hockey people. Even those who did use the books failed to understand his teachings as a philosophy and a holistic unit. Therefore, the "prophet without honour" and "genius we overlooked" tags are most applicable when looking at Percival's difficult relationship with Canada's favourite sport. Percival, however, rejected these labels, believing that his message had gotten through to at least some of the millions of people who had listened to "Sports College" and read the publications as well as to those thousands who read *The Hockey Handbook*.

Percival's impact on the coaching of junior age players was probably greater in the United States than it was in Canada. Since American players at that time had no illusions of one day playing in the NHL, they were less influenced by the NHL style of play, and their coaches were not constrained by the model imposed by the league. Johny Wilson at Princeton, Ned Harkness at RPI and Cornell and Lou Lamoriello at Providence College are only a few of the coaches who used *The Hockey Handbook* to bring about a renaissance in American hockey. By the time an organized coaching

---

1 Throughout these pages, the term "hockey" refers exclusively to men's hockey. When Percival produced his instruction books in the 1940s and 1950s, women's hockey was virtually extinct in Canada. A rebirth began in the 1960s and one of the pioneers, Harold Ribson, used *The Hockey Handbook* to introduce what he thought were Russian methods (*G&M* 14 Feb. 1969, 30). Ribson's teams were extremely successful and one appeared on the Ed Sullivan television show.

program was established in the United States, Percival's influence was firmly entrenched. Lou Vairo, one of the most influential figures in the emergence of the United States as a major force in international hockey, leaned heavily on Percival's writings when he set up the national coaching program in 1978 because he says, "*The Hockey Handbook* was the first book on hockey I ever read" and "it was one of my bibles." When Americans and college-trained Canadians who graduated from this system began making it to the NHL, they brought with them a style of hockey learned from Lloyd Percival.

Unfortunately for Percival and for hockey, the NHL continued to control the game in Canada at all levels and with an iron fist. Even though young players and minor league coaches were influenced by Percival, they were influenced more by the dream of playing in the NHL. Watching "Hockey Night in Canada" taught them more about how they needed to play the game than did listening to "Sports College." In 1964, Percival had pronounced, "NHL players are the most primitively coached and trained of all major athletes, because," according to Percival, NHL owners and coaches suffered from "ostrich syndrome, heads in the sand as hockey passes them by." They pulled their collective heads out of the sand briefly during the Summit Series in 1972 but only long enough to see that "good enough" had, once again, proven to be "good enough" for the NHL. It would take more than a decade before real cracks appeared in the NHL armour.

Aspects of Percival's teaching seeped into the NHL through coaches like Harry Sinden, as well as former NHL coach of the year, Bobby Kromm, and Don Cherry, who both grew up listening to "Sports College." Like so many others in the NHL, Cherry doesn't agree with everything Percival said, but he used parts of *The Hockey Handbook* when he was coaching and still has his original copy of the book. There is also Clare Drake, who briefly coached the Edmonton Oilers and who mentored many of the best coaches in Canada, and fellow former Edmonton head coach and Canadian National Team coach, Dave King. Marc Crawford is a former NHL coach of the year and a Stanley Cup champion. His father, Floyd Crawford, a member of the Belleville McFarlands during the World Championships in Prague in 1958, coached for fifty years using *The Hockey Handbook* because he says it "is my Bible. I am a disciple of Lloyd Percival and I passed it on to my sons." Buffalo Sabres head coach, Ron Wilson, was coached by Lou Lamoriello at Providence. His father, Larry, and his Uncle Johny were "Sports College" disciples and both coached in the NHL. Jim Rutherford, General Manager of the Stanley Cup Champion Carolina Hurricanes, trained under Percival at The Fitness Institute in 1970 and 1971, and the Hurricanes head trainer, Peter Friesen, who was presented with a copy of Percival's book by Dave King in 1980, wrote in 2006:

> I believe *The Hockey Handbook* written by Lloyd
> Percival and first published in 1951, remains the
> authoritative source for hockey fundamentals. It
> is my view that the training regimes that Percival
> developed based on those fundamentals have stood
> the test of time.

Still, this was not enough to change the culture of the NHL. As so often happens to Canadians who cannot find acceptance at home, Percival's formula for successful modern hockey had to be transported to other hockey playing nations before it could come back and be fully accepted in Canada. The first European player to have a significant impact on the NHL was Borje Salming who joined the Toronto Maple Leafs in 1973. The following year, the Winnipeg Jets of the new WHA built an international team around Bobby Hull and thrilled the fans with a fast and fluid international style – a "Percival style of play" according to Jets coach, Bobby Kromm, who said that Percival was the only coach who had "a significant impact" on him. It was not until the merger of the two leagues in 1980, followed by another period of expansion and the opening of the gates to a flood of Swedes and Finns that the culture of the NHL really began to change. After the first Russians, Czechs and Slovaks were officially allowed to emigrate in 1989, the NHL could no longer hold back time.

The simple presence of Russian, European and college-trained Americans in the NHL changed the way hockey is practiced and played in North America. The fitter and faster newcomers threatened the livelihood of every NHL player and any young player who one day hoped to make the grade. For the first time in NHL history, it was not an option that players train during the summer. Teams hired real trainers, and although there was nothing remotely resembling the kind of integrated system Percival had tried to introduce to professional hockey, more and more of the pieces of his system were becoming part of the NHL including the hiring of assistant coaches to teach specific aspects of the game as Percival had first suggested in 1944. Wayne Gretzky and Mario Lemieux helped disguise the situation for a while, but it eventually became clear that, with a few exceptions, the most skilled players in the NHL – and the most exciting – were Europeans and Russians. Sportswriters and fans wanted to know why the greatest hockey playing country in the world was not producing the greatest players. When the 2002 Olympics showcased a dazzling display of hockey talent and Team Canada proved that the best players in Canada could play this brand of hockey and still be the best in the world, fans were left wondering why they weren't able to watch this kind of hockey week after week and some of the players began to question the style and quality of the game in the NHL.

In 2005, players and management finally accepted that something had to be done about the way hockey was being played in the NHL. Some rules were changed and others were reinterpreted. The result is "the New NHL." It's still far from perfect – serious issues regarding interference and the acceptable level and form of violence in the game have to be resolved. In some ways, it still falls short of what Percival outlined in his training program for the 1950 Detroit Red Wings. However, the excitement generated by the speed and fitness of the men who now play the game is undeniable. What has so far gone unnoticed is that without Lloyd Percival and *The Hockey Handbook*, we probably would not have come this far.

Imagine that the American, Russian and the European hockey coaches had not read Percival's book and had only the NHL to look to for a model of hockey development. They would have adopted a variation on the style of hockey played in the NHL and Europeans, Russians and Americans who flooded the ranks of NHL teams in the 1980s and 1990s would have been trained in the same lackadaisical manner and indoctrinated with the same "dump, chase and hammer" mentality that dominated professional hockey in North America for decades. The NHL brain trust would simply have carried on as before, and the game would have become even more deeply inbred. Only because the new players had learned an alternative brand of hockey, hockey played the way Lloyd Percival taught it, hockey that is faster, more skilled and more interesting, was there impetus for change in the NHL. When the *Globe and Mail* pronounced in 2008, "The NHL game is full of it: Speed. Pace. Up Tempo. Quickness. ... hockey at the highest level has never been played with more swiftness," it confirmed that the NHL had finally caught up to Percival and his 1972 plan for the Detroit Red Wings to adopt "a performance tempo never achieved in hockey, of any classification." Lloyd Percival has been called the "stepfather of Russian hockey." He should also be recognized as "Father of the New NHL."

Coaching

A T SIXTEEN YEARS OF AGE, Lloyd Percival decided to become a coach and no matter what else he accomplished during his lifetime, it was his legacy as a coach that best defines him. No other Canadian coach of his era can claim anything close to the number of medals, trophies, championships and national records won by athletes he coached. No other coach affected the training of as many Olympians, and no other coach had as profound an influence on both amateur and professional athletes. Given the range of athletes and the variety of sports Percival touched, it is doubtful that anyone ever will. Because so many of his athletes became coaches themselves and inspired others to excel and to become coaches, Percival's contribution was exponential and continues to be felt today.

Within the fraternity of great coaches, there is a small cadre that are also great innovators. Percival sits at the head of the class. So many of the technical, physiological and psychological aspects of athletic training that Canadian coaches and athletes today take for granted were unheard of before Percival appeared on the scene. Through extensive research and the application of modern science, he made an enormous contribution to the growth and development of a number of sports in Canada and "goaded everybody into doing a better job." Sadly, so many of Canada's administrators, coaches and physical educators disliked Percival's aggressive approach, resented the way he accepted the status of "high priest" granted him by the media, and were jealous that he was able to make coaching his full-time job. In spite of the fact that he was posthumously inducted into Canada's Sports Hall of Fame, as well as the Canadian Boxing Hall of Fame and, in 2013, will take his rightful place in the Athletics Canada Hall of Fame (track and field), Percival has never received the recognition he deserves.

Percival is also the only coach in Canadian history who coached the entire nation. At a time when there was no other central source for coaching information and precious little informed coaching of any kind outside of the large urban centres, "Sports College of the Air" was informing young people in every corner of the country on the basics of healthy, athletic endeavour and sportsmanship. It is doubtful anyone aspiring to be a competitive athlete was unaware of the "Sports College" and countless young Canadians rarely missed a broadcast. Douglas Fisher was one of them. So was future national track and field coach, Andy Higgins, and countless future NHL players and coaches, including Derek Sanderson and Don Cherry who remembers vividly, "Every Saturday at 12:15 when we were young lads my mother made sausages and toast for my brother and me and we listened to "Ace" Percival on "Sports College." There is no way to even estimate the full impact of Percival's radio broadcasts and publications between 1944 and 1961, when "Sports College" spent more time and money on the promotion of fitness and sport than did the federal government, but Douglas Fisher called it "the untold story... the unbelievable reach and permeation of kids."

As with all good coaches, Percival's impact on the young people he coached, as well as those who listened to his radio broadcasts, reached beyond the fields and rinks where sport is played. It was the positive influence Percival exerted on their lives as adults that the men and women who trained under Percival remember most fondly. Peter Burwash who has achieved great success as an athlete, as a coach and as a motivational speaker testified before an Indiana State Commission on mandatory physical education in schools that the word "compete" comes from the Latin *com petere*, which means "to come together." This is a life lesson Percival attempted to impart to everyone he came in contact with or influenced through his writings, interviews and broadcasts. In a CBC radio interview, just months prior to his death, Percival discussed the modern dilemma of "competition" and his distress that it was becoming "a dirty word." He talked about how winning and losing were both important experiences in life and how the job of the coach was to teach athletes how to compete, how to win and how to lose, how to prepare for both and how to learn from both.

In spite of the range and depth of his contributions to Canadian sport and society, Percival often told people that he just wanted to be known as a coach. In light of the wide range of projects he initiated and the self-promotion in which he wrapped them, this might appear ingenuous and considering the list of achievements and contributions laid out in these pages, it seems like meagre homage. But it was something that Percival embraced when he was a teenager studying under Knute Rockne. Near the end of his life, Percival was still talking about the lessons he learned at the feet of his first mentor, how it was Rockne's "enthusiasm," "his tremendous zest and love of doing" which had impressed Percival most. Percival declared, "My ability to transmit that sort of zest is the key to any success I've had."

Epilogue

If Lloyd Percival were to come back to check up on "Mr. 2000," he would find sixty year old triathletes with abs of steel walking beside obese thirty year olds with type two diabetes; he would watch television highlights of two of the NHL's superstars, Canadian Sydney Crosby and Russian Evgeni Malkin, combining on as beautiful a goal as the NHL has ever seen, followed by a replay of the latest star player to suffer a concussion due to a vicious blow to the head; he would see a health club in every other suburban plaza, each flanked by fast food outlets; he would read about Canadian athletes winning more gold medals in Vancouver than any nation had won in any previous Olympics and Canada's summer athletes winning only one gold medal in London; and he would learn that baby yoga classes and kinder gyms are springing up everywhere even though so many of our children are overweight and morbidly obese that theirs will be the first generation in history to have a shorter lifespan than their parents.

Percival would probably be both honoured and disheartened by what he witnessed, but one thing is certain. He would immediately call a press conference and announce plans for improving the lot of "Mr. 2020."

Acknowledgements

This book required a number of years to progress from planning to interviews, to the page and finally to print. Without the generosity and patience of a great many people who shared a belief that the story of Lloyd Percival's life is important to Canadians, this book would never have been finished. Given the length of time since most of the interviews were conducted, we have been diminished by the passing of a number of significant contributors. The list includes: Joel Aldred; Bob Attersley; Wren Blair; Al Balding; Bill Dineen; Ron Dussiaulme; George Finlayson; Douglas Fisher; Trent Frayne; Murray Gaziuk; George Gross; Ned Harkness; Bobby Kromm; Ken Lane; Alyce MacLennan; Max McNab; Ron Miller; Gary Schreider; Joe Taylor; Johnny Wilson and John Wood.

I am especially grateful to Doug Fisher and Joe Taylor. Doug Fisher's understanding of Percival's critical role in the evolution of government policy for sport in Canada shed light upon an aspect of Percival's career that is little known. In addition, it was both Fisher's and Robert Fulford's insights into Percival's place in the cultural history of Canada which provided the framework for this biography. Joe Taylor, as well as Doug MacLennan, supplied much of the archival material used to piece together Percival's story. Along with John Hudson and Bill Gairdner, they provided important insights into Percival's life and work. Doug MacLennan also provided me with meticulous editorial assistance. Of course none of this would have meant anything if not for Dorothy and Jan Percival, who both allowed me into the private world of Lloyd Percival and trusted me to tell his story.

The list of people who also shared with me their memories of Lloyd Percival includes: Don Aitken; George Anthony; George Athans Jr.; Dave Bailey; John Bales; Sandra and Val Bezic; Tudor Bompa; Beverly Boys; Scotty Bowman; Charlie Bray; Ludek Bukac; Dr. Charles Bull; Bob Bursach; Peter Burwash; Leo Cahill; Paul Cerre; Margaret Cerre; Don Cherry; George Chuvalo; Dr. Doug Clement; Murray Cockburn; Murray Costello; Lee Coyne; Toller Cranston; Floyd Crawford; Judy Crawford (Rawley); Bill Crothers; Eddie Creed; Jack Creed; Gord Crosby; Clare Drake; Dave Dryden; Ken Dryden; Dick Duff; Alan Eagleson; Shirley Eckle(Kerr); Ron Ellis; Harry Fauquier; Peter Friesen; Greg Franke; Bill Gelling; Geoff Gowan, John Grant; Nancy Greene (Raine); Mort Greenberg; Bill Hay; Bill Heikilla; Andy Higgins; Derek Holmes; Gordie Howe; Jim Hunter; Dick Irvin Jr.; Dr. Roger Jackson; Rick Johnson; Jim Josephson; Dr. Terry Kavanagh; Red Kelly; Hermann Kerckoff; John Kernaghan; Bruce Kidd; Dave King; George Kingston; Russ Kisby; Murray Koffler; Seva Kukushkin; Chris Lang; Mary Lawrence; Nick Libbet; Ted Lindsay; Jocelyn Lovell; Bill Macdonald: Roy MacSkimming: Karen Magnussen; Frank Mahovlich; Dick Mathieu; Nancy McCredie; Jackie McDonald (Gelling); Brian McFarlane; Jack McRoberts; Wink McRoberts (Rogers); Bob Meldrum; Eleanor Miller; Don Morrow; Jim Mossman; Wayne Mullins; Eric Nestorenko; Emma Obodiac; Dean Oldershaw; John Panabaker; Peter Percival; Ivan Pintharic; Steve Podborski; Paul Poce; Bob Pulford; Clarke Pulford; Dan Pugilese; Pat Quinn; Al Raine; Nancy Robertson (Brawley); Lorne Rubenstein; Jim Rutherford; Larry Sadler; Bill Salter; Alan Scott; Isadore Sharpe; Dr. Roy Shephard; James Sinclair; Harry Sinden; Michael A. Smith; Jim and Marian Snyder; Al Sokol; Dave Steen; Stan Stiopkin; Alexey Tarasov; Charles 'Chuck' Tobias; Dr. Thomas Tutko; Irving Ungerman; Debbie Van Kiekebelt; Lou Vairo; Kevin Walmsey; Ron Wallingford; Terry Walker: Tom Watt; Don Webb: John Wildman; Ron Wilson; Jenny Wingerson (Madill) and Marvin Zucker.

Archivists are essential to the writing of any historical work, and I was fortunate to have the support of Miragh Addis at the Hockey Hall of Fame Archives, Brent Michaleff at the CBC Archives and Darren Yearsley at the CBC Licensing Division, Ian Fleming at the Y.M.C.A. Archives, Richard McQuade at St. Michael's College High School Archives and the always helpful staff at Library and Archives Canada. The historical pages of the Globe and Mail and the Toronto Star were scoured for innumerable columns and editorials related to Percival. In addition, the published works of the many and varied authors and journalists who have chronicled the remarkable times in which Percival lived have helped shape this book

No matter how much help you have in writing a book, an author must find people who have enough faith in the final product to bring it to the market. My agent, Peter Taylor, was the first to see the potential in this book and the first to search for a publisher with the same vision. It fell to Maureen Whyte at Seraphim Editions, however, to take a chance on an unproven author with a biography of a man who had been forgotten by Canadians, to understand that this is a story Canadians need to know and to shepherd this book until it came to life. My editor, Kathryn McKeen, has done a wonderful job of protecting me from myself and of presenting to the reader a book that is pleasing to the ear, while Julie McNeil has created an inspired cover and designed a book that is pleasing to the eye.

Gary Mossman is a freelance writer with a focus on history and sport. He is a member of the Society for International Hockey Research and has been published in *The Hockey News*. His book, *Fifty Years at the Royal Ashburn Golf Club*, was published in 2012. A biography of Father David Bauer, the Basilian priest 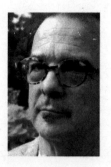 who coached Canada's National Hockey Team in the 1960s, is awaiting publication.

Gary Mossman lives in Toronto.